Belonging After Brain Injury

Belonging After Brain Injury: Relocating Dan explores the life of the author's brother who has dealt with the effects of a severe traumatic brain injury (TBI) for over four decades. It recounts the institutional, psychological, and social labyrinths he and his family have navigated following the TBI he sustained at the age of eighteen.

This insightful volume offers a holistic account of the impact of TBI on the survivor and his family. It reveals the difficulties a TBI survivor has had to endure and provides practical information about physical, psychological, and psychosocial symptoms and their consequences. Dan's story offers new perspectives and strategies that will help alleviate seemingly intractable problems and highlights the central importance of forming connections with others in order to lead a fuller life. The author's account of her own journey, learning to help care for her brother and advocate for him, offers an invaluable guide for TBI survivors and those who care for and support them.

Belonging After Brain Injury: Relocating Dan will be of interest to TBI survivors and their families. Its rich insights will be essential reading for medical and mental health professionals, as well as those involved in the care and rehabilitation of TBI survivors and families.

Katie H. Williams is a writer who formerly taught classes in cultural and interpersonal communication, rhetoric, and writing at Indiana University and Ivy Tech Community College. She is also Dan's sister who has made, and watched others make, mistakes over the past forty-three years that compromised the quality of his life, simply because she, and they, didn't know better. She learned a lot about these mistakes in her postgraduate education, studying communication and its impact on social as well as personal identity and belongingness. Then she learned more in the writing of this book, which she has put into practice with a satisfying degree of success.

After Brain Injury: Survivor Stories
Series Editor: Barbara A. Wilson

This new series of books is aimed at those who have suffered a brain injury, and their families and carers. Each book focuses on a different condition, such as face blindness, amnesia and neglect, or diagnosis, such as encephalitis and locked-in syndrome, resulting from brain injury. Readers will learn about life before the brain injury, the early days of diagnosis, the effects of the brain injury, the process of rehabilitation, and life now. Alongside this personal perspective, professional commentary is also provided by a specialist in neuropsychological rehabilitation, making the books relevant for professionals working in rehabilitation such as psychologists, speech and language therapists, occupational therapists, social workers and rehabilitation doctors. They will also appeal to clinical psychology trainees and undergraduate and graduate students in neuropsychology, rehabilitation science, and related courses who value the case study approach.

With this series, we also hope to help expand awareness of brain injury and its consequences. The World Health Organization has recently acknowledged the need to raise the profile of mental health issues (with the WHO Mental Health Action Plan 2013–20) and we believe there needs to be a similar focus on psychological, neurological and behavioural issues caused by brain disorder, and a deeper understanding of the importance of rehabilitation support. Giving a voice to these survivors of brain injury is a step in the right direction.

Published titles:

Reconstructing Identity After Brain Injury
A search for hope and optimism after maxillofacial and neurosurgery
Stijn Geerinck

Belonging After Brain Injury
Relocating Dan
Katie H. Williams

For more information about this series, please visit: www.routledge.com/After-Brain-Injury-Survivor-Stories/book-series/ABI

Belonging After Brain Injury
Relocating Dan

Katie H. Williams

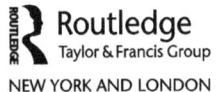

NEW YORK AND LONDON

Cover image: Getty Images

First published 2023
by Routledge
605 Third Avenue, New York, NY 10158

and by Routledge
4 Park Square, Milton Park, Abingdon, Oxon, OX14 4RN

Routledge is an imprint of the Taylor & Francis Group, an informa business

© 2023 Katie H. Williams

The right of Katie H. Williams to be identified as author of this work has been asserted in accordance with sections 77 and 78 of the Copyright, Designs and Patents Act 1988.

All rights reserved. No part of this book may be reprinted or reproduced or utilised in any form or by any electronic, mechanical, or other means, now known or hereafter invented, including photocopying and recording, or in any information storage or retrieval system, without permission in writing from the publishers.

Trademark notice: Product or corporate names may be trademarks or registered trademarks, and are used only for identification and explanation without intent to infringe.

Library of Congress Cataloging-in-Publication Data
Names: Williams, Katherine Hicks, author.
Title: Belonging after brain injury : relocating Dan / Katie H. Williams.
Description: First edition. | New York, NY : Routledge, 2023. |
  Includes bibliographical references and index.
Identifiers: LCCN 2022027788 (print) | LCCN 2022027789 (ebook) |
  ISBN 9781032374451 (hardback) | ISBN 9781032374475 (paperback) |
  ISBN 9781003340294 (ebook)
Subjects: LCSH: Brain—Wounds and injuries—Patients—Biography. |
  Post-traumatic stress disorder—Patients—Biography. | Brain—
  Wounds and injuries—Patients—Family relationships. | Brain—
  Wounds and injuries—Patients—Rehabilitation.
Classification: LCC RC387.5 .W5445 2023 (print) | LCC RC387.5
  (ebook) | DDC 617.4/81044—dc23/eng/20220923
LC record available at https://lccn.loc.gov/2022027788
LC ebook record available at https://lccn.loc.gov/2022027789

ISBN: 978-1-032-37445-1 (hbk)
ISBN: 978-1-032-37447-5 (pbk)
ISBN: 978-1-003-34029-4 (ebk)

DOI: 10.4324/9781003340294

Typeset in Bembo
by Apex CoVantage, LLC

For Dan Hicks, with immense love and admiration.

Disclaimer: This is a work of nonfiction. No characters have been invented, and no events have been fabricated. However, the names of people (except for those of my family) and most institutions have been changed in order to protect privacy and to avoid potential harassment.

Contents

	Acknowledgments	viii
	Introduction	ix
1	Obtaining Consent	1
2	Correcting the Record	23
3	Dan's Life: 1960–1984	35
4	Dan's Life: 1984–2006	55
5	Life at Trinity Village: 2006–2017	72
6	Crossing the Rubicon	91
7	New Normal	103
8	Finding Agape	122
9	Newer Normal	146
10	The Power of Belongingness	167
11	Epilogue	186
	Bibliography	189
	Index	191

Acknowledgments

I was working on this book long before I thought of writing it, and it is not separate from the rest of my life, so I am grateful to many, many people for many, many reasons, some in ways I can't even pinpoint. Over the years, countless sources offered concepts, theories, and case studies that helped me work out ways first to assist my brother, and then to write about them. Along with the researchers, theorists, and scholars whom I reference in these pages, innumerable others have informed and sharpened my thinking in ways that helped me to develop the understanding I needed to help Dan and to offer what I have learned to others. Most notable in this group are professors who introduced me to the riches of their fields and generously shared their knowledge and expertise, particularly Chris Poulos at the University of North Carolina Greensboro, and Jane Goodman, Susan Seizer, and John Lucaites at Indiana University Bloomington.

I'm deeply thankful for my parents, Glen and Happy Hicks, and my brother Dave, who taught me the unbreakable quality of love from the moment I entered the world. I owe the utmost gratitude to my brother Dan, who enthusiastically embraced the idea of this book and trusted me to share his story with the world. Finally, my debt to my husband, Dyke Williams, is incalculable. He supported me in the writing of this book in a host of ways, not least by paying the bills and believing in me. Dyke, my life would be decidedly less joyous and immeasurably less satisfying without you. With you, it is boundless.

Introduction

Imagine:

You receive the phone call: there's been an accident. Your brother (sister/mother/father/son/daughter/husband/wife) is comatose in an ICU, and *if* he doesn't die from his injuries, he may never regain consciousness. The next few hours and days will be critical, and should he survive, the prognosis, to the extent there can be one at this point, is bleak.

You are stunned. The shock is so intense that you undergo an immediate shift in consciousness, immersed in a sea of surreality that allows you to float through the next few minutes, hours, days, weeks. The world *looks* different. Colors are different—at once more vivid and less penetrating. Meaningless shapes, figures, faces swim by, hardly registering. This strange ocean allows you to function. You need this surreality, and you know you need it. You thank your brain for the gift.

In the waters that allow you to swim through this new reality, you notify your boss that you need to use your vacation days, starting now. You pack a suitcase, not giving much thought to what goes in or doesn't; your mind is elsewhere, trying *not* to process the news you've received. Your older brother—the bearer of that unbelievably bad news—has booked two seats on a red-eye flight departing at 3:00 a.m. When you meet him at the airport, you lock eyes. You know he sees the same shock in your eyes that you see in his. In that instant, the confirmation flares through the surreality: the world *has* changed, and this new world is *not* all right. And then, like a flash, the tide washes over you again, because you need it.

It's a fact that many thousands of people receive such news each year. Still, this news punches into your life like a fist. It feels like an intensely singular blow—as though no one, anywhere, ever, has been slammed by such news before. And in a sense, it is. Because there's only one person in this world who is the person lying in that hospital bed, surrounded by blinking machines humming and pulsing to keep him alive. If *he* is lost, there is no other *him*. And that fact, in that moment, is the epitome of tragedy.

Now imagine:
He is you.

★ ★ ★

This is the story of my brother Dan. It's a story of love and its trials, failures, and triumphs; of the workings of rejection and acceptance, of ostracism and inclusion, of disconnection and connection, and of the mortal consequences that these actions and states generate. It's a story of almost unimaginable challenges, of equally almost unimaginable persistence, of one man's push to construct a life of dignity and delight against all odds, and of the various forces that worked against him and with him, on his behalf. It's a story of investing every shred of revived hope and will in an effort to create a satisfying place in a world that, for decades, had quashed every attempt to claim one. In the end, it's a story of hope and vision and regeneration, but only if we, both as a society and as individuals, understand and accept the role we play in offering (or denying) dignity and connection to those who need it—and if we learn to recognize the gifts they are able, willing, and even gladdened to give, when given the chance.

In 1978, at eighteen years old, Dan was one of roughly 500,000 Americans who that year survived a TBI severe enough to lead to hospitalization or death.[1] In 1999, an estimated 5.3 million Americans were living with permanent TBI-related disabilities, with an additional estimated 80,000 to 90,000 people added to the roster each year.[2] In 2019 alone, American hospitals admitted 611 TBI patients every day.[3] The most frequent causes of TBI in the United States are falls, vehicular accidents, and violent events (including assaults and suicides involving firearms, the leading cause of TBI fatalities),[4] along with occupational and recreational sports-related accidents. Additionally, the wars in Iraq and Afghanistan have significantly swelled the numbers. In fact, the Department of Defense has called TBI "one of the signature injuries" of both wars,[5] with military training and combat incidences accounting for nearly 314,000 TBIs.[6] (While it has been widely publicized that a number of veterans of these wars commit suicide, what I have not heard noted is that many of these vets were suffering from TBI-related disabilities as a result of their military service, so that a number of these suicides may well have involved, if were not a direct result of, brain injury.) Across the board in all cases of incidents involving brain injury, it seems likely that the numbers reflect more people suffering severe disabilities due in part to continual advances in medical technologies, as many injuries that would have proven fatal just a few years earlier are now survived. Such interventions result in fewer deaths and so in more, and more severely impaired, TBI survivors.

At the same time, research into the mechanics of TBI and its effects has expanded, increasing the body of professional knowledge about these injuries. The relatively new field of neuropsychology has produced fresh insights into their neurological and resultant psychological effects. Even though every brain injury is unique (because the particulars of the accident cause specific degrees of damage to discrete areas of the brain), there are nevertheless certain common difficulties in cognitive and behavioral functioning, in patterns and to extents that correspond with the severity of the injury, that TBI survivors are likely to experience. A more detailed understanding of brain injury has led to the identification of a complex of symptoms and syndromes that might even be considered "normal" effects of brain injury. (It's worth pointing out here that, until I began researching brain injury for this book, I was not aware of the nature of these problems; I was merely perplexed and frustrated by them. At the time of Dan's injury, much of what now is known about TBI had yet to be discovered. My experience suggests that, although there has been some progress, even now many people entrusted with the care of TBI survivors—including doctors, nurses, hospital and nursing home staff, government agency professionals, and family members—remain unaware of the specific ramifications that brain injury entails.)

Beyond the neurological problems that result from damage to the brain, moderate to severe TBI survivors often face another problem that can be even more devastating than the issues caused directly by the injury itself: social disconnection from others. Responses to survivors that compromise social integration have many variations that social psychologists have classified into distinct categories: ostracism, exclusion, rejection, and bullying. Alienation and a sense of isolation are likely consequences. The sudden and enduring dismissal of survivors, most of whom enjoyed a typical degree of inclusion before their accidents, constitutes a form of social wounding that is experienced as both existentially frightening and agonizingly painful. *Belongingness*, a term that suggests one's sense of mutual and compatible integration with others, is an essential human need, and a lack of acceptance within the social body is not just unpleasant; it can be—and in Dan's case, seems to have been—literally a matter of life and death.

For decades, Dan has faced challenges on numerous fronts, and his serious impairments prevent smoothly moving through daily life on a logistical level. But they have had an even more damaging effect: they have severely restricted his acceptance into the realm of social life. Upon meeting him, most people only see a man slumped in a wheelchair, drooling onto his shirt, unable to talk, walk, or fluidly move, and their common reactions have caused him more pain and hardship than any of the logistical obstacles he has had to work around. At various times, within various settings, to various degrees, and with variously severe repercussions, Dan has been denied full human status—not because people are evil or uncaring but because they couldn't perceive the fully human spirit locked within his compromised self-presentation. As a result, he has been all too often deprived of consideration as a person deserving of time, concern, and dignity in full measure, even as his impairments heighten his need of them. Dan is fully capable of relationship—of *mutual* relationship, that allows him the opportunity to give as well as receive—but, routinely, that capability has been underestimated or even completely overlooked. Consequently, he has often been deprived of what he (like everyone else) needs most: the certain assurance that he is known and considered worthy of concern and affiliation by those around him, that he is mutually connected to others who like or love him, others who are personally, intimately invested in whether he lives or dies and how well he does either. In a word, he needs *belonging*.

In the more than forty years since his accident, life for Dan has been a relentless quest to regain a sense of normalcy—intuited as the ground in which belongingness is rooted—and, failing that, a satisfactory level of dignity. Adjustment to his impairments continually took a back seat to his drive for restoration and so has been incremental, as the unrelenting seesaw between loss and rehabilitation has pushed him inexorably, excruciatingly further toward loss. I've never seen, and can't imagine, anyone in any circumstances exhibiting more grit than my brother. For me, he's the very model of courage, determination, resilience, and sheer, relentless persistence.

Elements of Dan's injury and its multiple effects will resonate with many TBI survivors, as well as with their families and care providers. While Dan's story is interesting in its own right, I hope (as does he) that by sharing it, survivors may find a sense of camaraderie, inspiration, and perhaps increased self-acceptance. I especially hope that at least some families and care providers will gain more understanding of the sometimes exasperating, mystifying, and even self-defeating perspectives and behaviors that survivors may exhibit. While understanding problems is not the same as resolving them, understanding often can reduce the angst and anger that otherwise might seize others in their presence, driving wedges that further separate survivors from the most important people in their lives. There is no *cure* for TBI, but the problems it causes often can be made better or worse—for everyone involved—depending on the degree of insight we can apply when we experience them.

★ ★ ★

Dan's story is also an integral part of my own story. Words can't adequately express the pain I (and the rest of my family) experienced from Dan's accident. The intensity of that pain never waned, and unfortunately, and to my shame and deep regret, I dealt with it by separating myself from him, on some level believing that if I got too close, the pain would swallow me whole. At first, it *did*. Seven months after Dan's TBI, I dropped my college classes and joined the Navy in an attempt to halt my spiraling anger and despair. I never stopped loving Dan—indeed, it was my love for him (and probably a hefty measure of survivor's guilt) that made it so difficult to make peace with his accident and its aftermath; but for years I mostly hovered about the margins of his life, afraid to completely enter his reality or allow him to enter mine. In truth, below conscious awareness, I viewed Dan's postaccident life as a crushing black hole. I performed my role as the dutiful sister, and while the performance was heartfelt—often painfully so—it was also forced. In ways neither my family nor I realized, I wrapped myself in a blanket of distance, despite love's tremendous gravitational pull.

In sum, for years I experienced Dan's postaccident life as an unmitigated catastrophe. It wasn't until decades later—until soon after the story as I have written it here begins—that I realized that Dan is not, and never was, a tragedy. Neither he nor his life is deficient or hopelessly broken. Regarding him now, I am reminded of *kintsugi*, a Japanese method of mending broken pots by joining their fragments with lacquer and powdered gold or other precious metals. This process conceives of reconstitution as an art form, through which the gleaming "scars" left by the breaking bestow unique character and singular beauty to the piece made whole again—never the same, but artfully whole.

Dan has endured immeasurably more than his share of adversity, and he has taught me an invaluable lesson: approached with the right spirit, a refusal to crumble, and assurance of mutual connectedness, adversity and exuberance can coexist. Dan's life is as full, and even as happy, as anyone's I know. And entering his orbit—becoming a genuine part of his life—has been an unexpected joy for me. Dan's story is also, then, a story of my own awakening to the gifts my brother brings me, not least of all to the delight that comes from sharing our non-negotiable, bone-deep connectedness. And I hope that telling this story might foster similar awakenings in families and various care providers across the country.

★ ★ ★

A brief explanation of the sources I used to reconstruct Dan's life history:

I utilized what I personally know of Dan and his life, informed by my own memories and family stories circulated in the context of our lives together. This information was augmented by documents I gathered in 2002 to write my master's thesis. For that project, I consulted clinical records as well as correspondence between my parents (writing on Dan's behalf) and various organizations and agencies. At that time, I also engaged in extensive conversations with my mother and our brother Dave (my father was no longer living) to glean their memories and experiences. Additionally, for my thesis, in January 2003, Dan and I spent thirty-six hours exploring his thoughts, recollections, and feelings about his life up to that point.

In writing about the period between Dan's move from Taylor Heights Health and Rehabilitation Center in 2003 until he took up residence at Trinity Village in 2006, I have relied on my own experiences with him, conversations with my brothers, care provider records, and medical reports.

I documented Dan's life at Trinity Village using extensive notes detailing weekly (and at times more frequent) phone conversations I had with Dan. This ten-year electronic log began several months before he arrived at Trinity Village. I started keeping track of Dan's side of our conversations during our phone calls largely because visualizing the letters he typed on his Speak'n'Spell, a device he uses to give sound to individual letters (we hadn't yet developed our "alphabetting" system), assisted me in stringing together words and substituting correct letters when he mistyped or I misheard them. Also, I soon learned that referring to earlier notes helped me maintain conversational continuity from week to week, so I began to chronicle my side of the conversations too—my questions and observations, as well as his answers and comments. At the outset, I had no idea that these logs would form a comprehensive record of Dan's life at Trinity Village, from the first week he took up residence in May of 2006 until July of 2015, months after he was no longer able to communicate through his Speak'n'Spell. At that point, following months of entries noting only the briefest sketches of my comments, since he had virtually stopped responding, I stopped keeping any record of the now one-sided conversations.

Finally, in early 2017, several months after I began reading to Dan over the phone each day, and only months before beginning the process of bringing him to Indiana, I initiated a Dan-focused personal journal. I began simply by noting the titles of books I thought might interest him (riveting works that center around horse racing are neither plentiful nor easy to obtain), but the journal expanded as I began adding my impressions of the various nursing homes I looked into and of discussions related to the prospective move. As I began encountering hurdles, roadblocks, and nasty surprises, the journal became the repository of my frustrations, distress, and anger as well as of the details of events and conversations as they unfolded.

Writing the story of my brother's life by bringing together memories, conversations, family records, clinical reports, and a wide-ranging body of professional literature has been an inexpressibly gratifying experience. The life Dan led before his injury was shattered more than forty years ago. Over the years, he has carefully gathered the shards and found new ways to fit them together. His postaccident life is nowhere near perfect, but it glints at the seams. Both Dan and I hope that sharing his story will be useful to others who face similar challenges, and to those who care for them.

Notes

1. "Traumatic Brain Injury in the United States: A Report to Congress" *Centers for Disease Control and Prevention* (December 1999, 5). www.cdc.gov/traumaticbraininjury/pdf/TBI_in_the_US.pdf
2. "Report to Congress: Traumatic Brain Injury in the United States" *Centers for Disease Control and Prevention* (January 2016, 1). www.cdc.gov/traumaticbraininjury/pubs/tbi_report_to_congress.html
3. "TBI Data" *Centers for Disease Control and Prevention.* Centers for Disease Control and Prevention, March 21, 2022. www.cdc.gov/traumaticbraininjury/data/
4. "Get the Facts about TBI" *Centers for Disease Control and Prevention.* Centers for Disease Control and Prevention, March 21, 2022. www.cdc.gov/traumaticbraininjury/get_the_facts.html
5. "Traumatic Brain Injury: Department of Defense Special Report" *Legacy Homepage.* U.S. Department of Defense. https://dod.defense.gov/News/Special-Reports/0315_tbi/
6. "TBI Among Service Members and Veterans" *Centers for Disease Control and Prevention.* Centers for Disease Control and Prevention, July 26, 2022. www.cdc.gov/traumaticbraininjury/military/index.html

1 Obtaining Consent

August 13, 2017

We breezed into Dan's room, me clutching my laptop like a paramedic with a defibrillator. I couldn't see my brother's face, and he couldn't see my husband Dyke or me until we had crossed the room to his bedside.

"Hey, Dan!" I sounded cheery, but I was nervous. So much depended on this visit.

Dan lifted his arm in response, smiling big. He looked relaxed, even serene. Still, the arm he raised in welcome was weak and thin, his wrist bones and the slender muscle tethered to them stark in the fluorescent light.

After some lighthearted chatter, I phoned in an order to Five Guys, and Dyke left to pick it up. While we waited for the food, I offered a running stream of banter, with Dan murmuring in response to my comments and jokes, occasionally fingerspelling words to inject his own thoughts. When Dyke returned with Dan's double cheeseburger and mocha milkshake, I made a salad from the burger's add-ons—lettuce, tomato, pickles, and onion—and slathered it in ketchup, then delivered forkfuls to his mouth. His acceptance of my feeding him was as new as his decision to stay in bed four months earlier. Along with the more relaxed curve of his neck as he lay supine with the pillow cradling his head, my conveyance of the food made his eating more efficient—quicker and cleaner, with less food escaping his mouth—and more pleasant (for me, at least, and maybe for him too) than when he fed himself. Still, I didn't entirely welcome this new development. I wondered if, like his recent decision to stay in bed rather than to get up each day, abandoning his determination to eat unassisted signaled resignation. An end of sorts.

This visit would deviate from our customary pattern. Usually, Dyke's and my trips from Indiana to Georgia were quick weekend jaunts. On Friday after work, we'd drive from our home in Fishers until about one

DOI: 10.4324/9781003340294-1

in the morning, spending the rest of the night at a Sleep Inn in central Tennessee. Saturday morning we'd start the route to Metro Atlanta. By midday, we'd arrive at Trinity Village, the nursing home where Dan lived, take him out to an early dinner, and, after spending the night at the local Days Inn, return to Indiana on Sunday. This current visit would break the form. Instead of following our usual itinerary, Dyke would be driving back to Fishers by himself the next day while I stayed at Trinity Village for three days more, when I would take a plane back to Indianapolis. This visit would give me more time to conduct my mission.

And so as I fed Dan, keeping up a steady patter of small talk, I bided my time, awaiting the right moment to deliver my presentation. Tomorrow would be a better time for it, I thought. I wanted a leisurely conversation, with both of us relaxed and well-rested. So much depended on the upcoming discussion. In fact, although I didn't realize it at the time, Dan's life literally hung in the balance.

★ ★ ★

A lot had happened in the previous three weeks, beginning with Dyke's and my visit with Dan in late July.

First, I learned the real reason for Dan's decision in April to remain in bed permanently. When my brother Dave told me that Dan no longer wished to get up, I was alarmed. Dave and I discussed Dan's decision over the phone. Dan was getting older (he had just turned fifty-seven), and Dave, a retired medical corpsman in the Navy, told me that decades of living with TBI accelerates the aging process. Dan was, he surmised, physically and emotionally spent, no longer having the energy to engage the daily struggle life had been requiring of him for years. As Dave put it, Dan had "squeezed out all the juice" that life could offer him, and we were witnessing his inevitable decline. Along with his years of medical experience, Dave had been a continual presence in Dan's life for years and knew him better than anyone else on the planet, including me, so I figured he must be right. Reflecting on our conversation that evening, I wrote in my journal, "If we measure our lives by how much we get out of them, how much there is to get, Dan's had to fight for every ounce, and it's hard to see where any more juice might be." I ended the entry with, "I feel like I'm writing an elegy." No wonder Dan had given up, I thought.

Further stoking what Dave and I assumed was a case of sheer fatigue, Dave had just moved from Georgia to Maryland—like Indiana, ten hours away by car. For years, Dave had been Dan's most active support. I spoke with Dan every day, and I read to him each night on the phone, but I lived in Indiana. Dyke and I only visited every few months. Dave visited

Dan each week, taking him out for lunch at Hooters, or sometimes to a strip club or a movie. They occasionally took more extensive trips too, although, because of Dan's physical decline, it had been a while since the last one. When Dan decided to stay in bed three months earlier, Dave's weekly visits became eat-ins in Dan's room, with Dave bringing in pizza or cheeseburgers. Following Dave's recent move to Maryland, Dan was surely feeling the absence of his brother, who was also his closest friend. It was understandable that he'd be depressed.

But when I saw him in July, Dan didn't look depressed. In fact, he looked younger and less stressed than he had in years. Paradoxically, I thought, giving up on life seemed to have been restorative. But when I asked him why he had decided to remain bed-bound, Dan spelled "SORE." He wasn't world-weary, fatigued, and depressed. The simple fact was that getting up and moving around had become painful. When he weighed costs and benefits, he determined that the marginal satisfactions he derived from dressing, moving from bed to wheelchair, sitting all day, and then undressing for bed were outweighed by their cost in pain. Besides, he noted, when he was lying on his back, eating and toileting were easier, and he remained cleaner. Clearly the change had relieved him; he looked fifteen years younger than he had on our visit a few months earlier. I was flabbergasted that both Dave and I had so misread the situation, and that, in the wake of our assumptions, neither of us had ever asked Dan about it.

The visit in July also taught me that the pressure sores which had begun developing on Dan's hip and heels were not a result of what the wound nurse had termed "resistance" to her advice. She had reported to me that she had recommended that he periodically shift his weight to remove pressure on the affected areas, but he was refusing to do it. Because Dan had struggled mightily off and on for several years with a pressure sore at the base of his spine, I couldn't understand why he would willfully incur additional sores in new places. So I figured I'd reason with him on our July visit and try to get him to follow the nurse's guidance. He surprised me by agreeing that the nurse's recommendation was sound—indeed he fervently wished he could comply with it. Unfortunately, he conveyed to me, he was physically unable to shift his weight in bed. Thinking that maybe I could request that Trinity Village's staff help him turn onto his side for a while each day, to allow blood to circulate into the compressed areas of his hip and heels, I tried to help him alter his position. I was gentle, and he is as tough as men come, but he gasped and winced with pain. He could no longer comfortably move, period.

I wondered then, aloud, how many times Dan's behavior had been chalked up to refusal out of stubbornness and resistance when the "refusal" was actually inability. He repeatedly flexed the fingers of his left hand, his gesture for "innumerable."

I asked Dan what he did all day, lying motionless in bed. He spelled "CEILING"; because he couldn't even angle himself into a position that allowed him to watch the TV on his dresser a few feet away, he listened to ESPN while staring at the ceiling. "It sounds like you're bored a lot," I said, and he emphatically nodded.

I noted on this visit the extreme importance of small details to someone in Dan's position. For example, a desk clock within his line of sight had lost power weeks before, and the LED display had been flashing ever since. Dyke noticed and reset the clock, and Dan seemed inordinately pleased. When I later mentioned it to Dave, he asked if Dan was wearing his watch. He was. But he was vexed by that blinking clock—not because he didn't know what time it was but because the clock had been serving no purpose other than to remind him of his inability to reset it. Similarly, I unraveled the cord on his telephone, which had twisted into a ball, tremendously shortening its reach. Having it unwound was a big deal to him—another one of those little irritants that he could do nothing about. I asked him if anything else was bothering him, and he answered that his TV Guide subscription was about to lapse, and he didn't have fresh batteries for his TV remote—concerns that I could easily address but Dan couldn't. I pledged to take care of those problems, and he smiled, relieved.

That July visit also initiated a major development in both Dan's and my lives: with Dave no longer living in the area, Dan and I discussed the possibility of his moving to Indiana to be near family—to be near me. I made it clear that I understood that whether or not he moved was 100 percent his choice, and I promised I wouldn't try to pressure him. And I meant it. I comprehended the enormity of such a decision for someone in his position. Although he was unable to speak and hardly able to move, I was asking him to relocate to a new facility in a part of the country he had never visited, surrounded by people he didn't know and couldn't talk to—to be reliant upon these strangers for helping him with the minutest, most intimate and essential tasks of his daily life. His situation at Trinity Village was not pleasant, but it was at least familiar, and that familiarity hadn't developed overnight. Turning strangers into familiar faces, even if some were not friendly, had taken considerable time. I knew the idea of uprooting from the place he'd lived for eleven years was daunting, but with Dave no longer nearby, Dan was now 600 miles away from both of us, what remained our family. I assured Dan that I wasn't just willing to take on a more active role in his life but that I genuinely wanted to. If he agreed to relocate, I said, I vowed to do everything in my power to make the transition as smooth as possible and to improve his quality of life as much as possible. I acknowledged that I didn't have much of a record to point to that would give him confidence in me—I had hovered on the periphery of his life for years, only occasionally stepping in deeper to intervene when I felt I was needed—but I pledged that he could count on me. In response, Dan eyed me dubiously and spelled "GOOD": he was open to the idea of moving to Indiana if I could find a place that was good. I assured him that my aim was to improve his situation, not worsen it, and I swore I wouldn't move him unless I was confident that his life would be better as a result.

Spurred by this conversation, my search for a good nursing home in Indiana escalated from an online theoretical exercise to a boots-on-the-ground quest for a new home for my brother.

★ ★ ★

I'm habitually on the lookout for real-life metaphors, and I hoped that the hailstorm I was driving into on my way to visit nursing homes in Muncie wasn't one of them. But then I extended the metaphor, upending it: I was successfully pushing through the pelting hail as I splashed across the Indiana landscape, determined to find good shelter from the storm for Dan.

Indianapolis offered many more long-term care facilities than Muncie, and it was considerably closer to Dyke's and my home in Fishers, but we were already in the process of house-hunting in Muncie. I wanted to be able to view visits with Dan as quick jaunts across town that I could make on the spur of the moment as wanted or needed, so proximity was a major consideration. I had three Muncie nursing homes on my list that day, all of which rated highly according to *US News & World's Report* online. I was leery of touring the facilities with someone hired for the purpose of recruiting residents, so I was hoping to at least superficially explore them unannounced in order to get a sense of what living in them might be like.

The first facility had the feel of a cushy four-star hotel: decorative tile, gleaming wood, soft lighting. But I never got beyond the front desk. Only ten of sixty-eight beds were reserved for Medicaid recipients, the desk attendant told me, and not only were those beds full but the waiting list was already prohibitively long. And had I only imagined her dismissive sniff when I mentioned Medicaid? The entire visit lasted less than five minutes.

Discouraged but not daunted, I went to the second place on my list. There was no sniffing when I asked about Medicaid, but I again didn't get past the front desk. When I noted that Dan was currently in a Georgia facility, I was directed downtown to file appropriate paperwork with the

Division of Family Resources, which would help me arrange an interstate transfer of his Medicaid, provided Dan was eligible. Once his status had been approved, I could return for a tour. I answered that I would check into it and get back with them, but I added internally, "only as a last resort."

When I entered the third and last facility on my list, the front desk was unattended, so I walked through the reception area up to a nurse's desk, also unattended. Lights were flashing, and the desk was sparsely littered with half-empty cups of orange juice and vanilla pudding. I waited a few minutes and was about to leave when someone surfaced from one of the hallways, asking, "Can I help you?" I stated my business and was led to an office where an earnest young woman interviewed me. She scribbled details of my inquiry into a notebook, indicated that she would take care of any necessary paperwork to transfer Dan's Medicaid, and took me on a brief tour. The facility appeared to be in generally good shape, but an undercurrent of feces and urine permeated the air, hardly noticeable in some areas but pungent in others. I took the proffered literature and left, feeling that I had lost this day's battles but secure in the faith that I'd win the war.

A few days later, I solicited recommendations at my church. The second facility I had visited the day of the hailstorm, Harbor Health of Muncie, resurfaced as a possibility. The friend who suggested it was surprised when I described my brief visit to Harbor as unimpressive and those at the front desk as discouragingly unhelpful. But my friend is a state representative with numerous connections and a comprehensive knowledge base of her district to draw from, so her opinion outweighed my first impression. She offered to connect me with Harbor's director, and a few days later I pulled into its parking lot with a tumultuous mix of hope, anxiety, and resolve. It was a tall order, but I was committed to finding a place that would offer Dan a better life than he currently had at Trinity Village. I was seeking, above all, a place where he not only would be safe but where he would feel at home.

★ ★ ★

I was a few minutes early for my appointment with Shiloh, Harbor Health's administrative director, and before I had finished reporting my arrival at the front desk, she emerged from her office with her hand already extended. "Katie?" she asked with a pleasant smile. She exuded an affable calm as she shook my hand and led me into her office, and I already felt more at ease.

Once we were seated, Shiloh asked me what had brought me to Harbor. I explained that since Dave's move a few weeks earlier, Dan was stranded without family in the Atlanta area, so I wanted to bring him to Indiana to live near me. "Family is so important," she agreed. "Tell me more about your brother."

I opened with what I assumed from her perspective she was most interested in knowing, and through a question-and-answer period, a picture of Dan emerged. In the aftermath of the TBI he sustained decades ago, I said, Dan has struggled with various severe impairments. He's paralyzed on his right side and uses a wheelchair. He has Broca's aphasia, which means his ability to formulate language is severely restricted, but he understands everything that is said to him. And, surreptitiously evaluating Shiloh's reaction, I explained that, as is common in people with a serious TBI, Dan has spasmodic bursts of rage that seem to arise from nowhere, although I conveyed my personal observation that they seem most likely to flare when he feels as though his competence is underestimated or his sense of autonomy is undermined. Shiloh nodded. The incidents typically pass quickly, I continued, although their duration can be extended when others react in ways that exacerbate his frustration. But even when they're brief, I admitted, these episodes are certainly impressive—and very unpleasant—while he is experiencing them.

"Is he violent during these times?" Shiloh asked, unruffled. Her evenness gave me hope.

"He can appear violent," I answered carefully, "but Dan's not an angry or violent person. He's usually pleasant to be around." I took a breath. "There was an incident at his current facility five years ago when someone felt threatened, but he's never actually hurt anyone."

I half expected Shiloh to eject me from her office after this piece of information. When she didn't, I asked her if she had time to hear more about Dan's history. I wanted to balance the roster of his deficits with a sketch of his life over the past years: how thoroughly his world had crashed in his late adolescence, how much sheer grit he had exhibited in fighting to restore his life, how relentlessly the losses had piled up, and how persistently he had rallied, over and over, to regain as much control over his life as he could. He struggled to recover as much normalcy as possible, striving to retain his dignity even when his compromised body or external circumstances sabotaged him. I wanted Shiloh to understand that Dan was not a pathetic, unwieldy, angry victim of tragedy but a warrior—imperfect, for sure, but nevertheless a courageous, indefatigable, battle-tested survivor.

I was grateful when Shiloh encouraged me to fill in whatever blanks I felt were important. She listened patiently, even intently, as I did:

In 1978, two weeks before his high school graduation, while Dan was working as an apprentice quarter horse trainer on a ranch in Oklahoma, he was kicked in the head by a horse. Hoof met skull, and in that fraction of a second, life as he'd known it ended. He was rushed to a Tulsa hospital, where his survival was in doubt as he hovered between life and death, and doctors refused to speculate on his odds of survival. After the first days, when it seemed increasingly likely that he would live, they were careful not to offer too much hope that he would ever regain consciousness. But after two months, he finally began to show the first small signs of emerging from the coma. Still barely and only intermittently conscious, Dan was transferred by air ambulance to Fullerton, the Southern California town where my parents lived, where he remained hospitalized for another six months. As he became more fully aware of himself and his surroundings, a gradual process that took several weeks, he found himself in a hospital bed with no recollection of either the accident or his hospital stay in Tulsa. His last clear memories were of life as a high school senior and expert horseman; when he awoke, he was breathing and being fed through tubes, and he was barely able to move a single toe or finger. And while he clearly understood what was said to him, he himself was unable to utter a word.

As months passed, Dan marshaled his strength and approached his rehabilitation with his characteristic optimism, vigor, determination, patience, and even good humor. He worked hard to relearn standing, walking, eating, toileting, and brushing his teeth—the countless activities most of us routinely perform every day as we take for granted the complex coordination of our movements, manipulating the physical world without much conscious thought. Dan's efforts were impressively successful; by July, he was able to independently eat, dress himself, take care of his personal grooming needs, and walk (if a bit unsteadily) with the assistance of a pair of four-pronged canes with braces that fit over his forearms. He was released from the hospital to continue therapy as an outpatient, returning to the same bedroom in our family home that he had left, under radically different circumstances, only a year earlier.

By October of 1979, three months after his release from the hospital, Dan already had formulated strategies to begin putting his life together—not the life he had expected the year before but one that was active, engaged, and as fully "normal" as he could make it. Although he had been awarded his high school diploma (in absentia, two weeks after the accident while he was still comatose), Dan wanted to work on sharpening the cognitive skills that his TBI had blunted, so he enrolled in a special program at a nearby high school. Because he still had serious problems with balance, he used a walker rather than the pronged canes he used at home. For additional safety, a classmate was assigned to accompany him from class to class. Despite these precautions, however, on his first day in the program, Dan lost his balance on a concrete walkway between school buildings and fell, shattering the cranial plate that, eleven months earlier, surgeons had inserted to replace the fragmented parts of his skull.

Much of the impairment Dan has lived with over the years has been a direct result of this second accident, from which he lost nearly all movement and feeling on his right side—arm, hand, leg, and foot. He is right-handed, so much of his earlier rehabilitation had focused on regaining the use of his right hand. Consequently, he had still relied on it—as most right-handed people do—to perform most tasks, such as eating, writing, and brushing his teeth. Because of this second accident, however, the tasks he had so painstakingly relearned with his right hand, he then had to learn to perform with his left—a difficult challenge for any right-handed person. Walking became more difficult too, because his right leg and foot, rather than serving as his main support, were now essentially dead weight. Over the next few years, he put his entire being into programs intended to restore the functions and skills he had lost, earning only scant returns on his immense physical and psychic investments. He was loath to concede permanence to any of his new impairments, no matter how obviously irremediable they were to others. For example, it required several years of concentrated urging from his family and therapeutic experts before he finally agreed to use a wheelchair.

When our parents relocated from California to Georgia in 1980, Dan moved with them. They built a studio apartment onto their house to give their son a measure of the independence he so craved as a twenty-year-old young adult, while still providing the assistance he needed. Still, Dan hungered for a more independent adulthood. In 1990, he signed a one-year lease with a government-subsidized assisted living complex in Savannah, an hour's drive from our parents' house, with the expectation of returning to his apartment in our parents' home at the end of the year.

As it turned out, Dan lived at Oliver Place for almost twelve years. His life in Savannah was solitary, but he gained the independence he desired and so was unwilling to relinquish it when the year was over. Not until July 2002 did the family discover just how challenging those years had been. One Saturday afternoon, Dan fell in his kitchen and spent hours on the floor, unable to reach either his wheelchair or the emergency call button on the wall. He hollered until he had no voice left, but no one heard him. The personal aide who was scheduled to help him exercise on Sunday mornings never showed up. Dan lay helpless on the floor until he was discovered by Oliver Place staff late Monday morning, unconscious, severely dehydrated, and in renal failure—in short, near death. He was rushed by ambulance to the emergency room and admitted into the hospital.

Dan survived, but X-rays revealed a number of old scars on his bones from fractures that had healed untreated. His physician suspected that he was the victim of severe, ongoing physical abuse until his vehement denials convinced her otherwise. We were horrified by the news that Dan had sustained fractures without telling anyone. Either Dan was unaware of the gravity of his injuries and so had never mentioned them or—more likely—he had not mentioned his injuries lest he be forced to abandon his independent life in Savannah.

But now Dan had no choice. The hospital doctor refused to release him to return to Oliver Place, which didn't much matter since the complex was unwilling to allow him to come back anyway; a certain level of self-sufficiency was required to live there, and it was clear that he no longer met their qualifications. Mom deeply regretted that she couldn't bring him home to live with her, but, since our father had recently died and she herself was debilitated by advancing emphysema, she simply couldn't manage the level of care he required. His options had suddenly telescoped.

Dave lived in an Atlanta suburb and scrambled to find a nearby nursing home with an open spot. When Dan was released from the hospital, he moved into Taylor Heights Health and Rehabilitation Center, close enough for Dave to make weekly visits. After the traumatic Oliver Place debacle, Mom, Dave, and I were relieved that Dan was safe, and we put the best face on it we could, encouraging him to adapt to this latest shift in his circumstances. But Dan was despondent, and no wonder. Nursing homes have an invaluable mission, as I was quick to acknowledge in my recounting of Dan's story to Shiloh, but these facilities are designed to satisfy the needs of two specific populations, neither of which Dan is a member: patients who need short-term physical therapy before returning to their homes, and elderly people approaching the end of their lives with chronic illnesses or dementia. Shiloh didn't take offense; rather, she agreed. For most people, she pointed out, "long-term" care at a nursing facility typically spans no more than a few years. But Dan, at only forty-two years old when he entered Taylor Heights, would likely live for decades—he was disabled, not ill—and she understood why the idea of spending the rest of his life in a nursing home would be utterly dispiriting. I continued with my account: in Taylor Heights, after twenty-four years of an intense, ceaseless struggle for autonomy and independence, Dan felt even more separated from the world of the fully living, which he had spent his entire adult life struggling to be part of, and which we were now encouraging him to give up hope of rejoining.

Four months after his move to Taylor Heights, I spent a week interviewing Dan for my master's thesis, which was a study of the impact of disability on identity. We both enjoyed the time we spent together, and Dan appreciated the opportunity to help me in my work as much as I appreciated his help. I got to know my brother much better. We discussed at length his life before and after the accident, exploring his memories as well as his thoughts and feelings about events and circumstances he had dealt with. That visit—a brief but intense immersion into his perspective—fostered in me a radical empathy for Dan and what this latest situation meant to him. He deeply resisted the idea of "adapting" to life in a nursing home, which he equated with a premature, painfully protracted death. While I worried that leaving the safety of Taylor Heights might not work out well for him, I worried more about the damage to his psychological health if he stayed. So at Dan's request and after sincerely apologetic discussions with Dave (who had worked hard to find a residence for Dan post-Oliver Place), I orchestrated, by phone from Indiana over a period of months, Dan's transfer from Taylor Heights into the agency-overseen private home of a human services care provider.

Dan experienced this move into a community setting as a reprieve, and initially the situation seemed to be working well. But before two years had passed, his ongoing problems with rage outbursts and his dismissal of some of the safety rules the care provider had established led to an abrupt, unceremonious end to the placement. He ended up living for a year in a couple's basement while inching upward on local nursing home waiting lists. The basement was well-appointed, and Dave visited each week, but following an accident with his wheelchair that damaged a piece of furniture, Dan's use of his wheelchair was banned, leaving him to spend the rest of the year sitting alone on a couch watching television. My efforts to get him out of Taylor Heights and into a community setting had been well-intentioned, but they had backfired. Dan still insists that he doesn't regret having tried the community placement, but the overall experience was sufficiently miserable that he was relieved when a bed finally opened up at Trinity Village, an hour's drive from Dave's house. Dan accepted, however reluctantly, that a nursing home was the best option available to him.

Shiloh was still listening to Dan's story with interest, so I elaborated a bit on the episode I had been most concerned about explaining. I told her that in December of 2012, one of the staff members at Trinity Village claimed that Dan had tried to "run her down" with his motorized wheelchair. He admitted to me that he intended to scare her—which was bad enough—but swore he would never have physically harmed her. "He doesn't lie," I said, "so I'm sure he believes that, but I don't know what the truth of the moment was. Her perceptions and his differ, and I wasn't there." Whatever the actual situation was, I continued, Dan was taken to

Cornerstone Hospital, a psychiatric facility, for a week of evaluation and observation. His agreement to take medication was a condition of returning to Trinity Village. The facility also put a speed-restricting governor on his wheelchair. But a few months later, the medicine was discontinued and the governor was removed. I added, "He's not had a similar problem since, although he does still have those flash anger episodes."

And so, I concluded, here I was at Harbor Health, seeking a nursing home in Muncie so that I could take Dave's place as Dan's point person—his family presence, his liaison, his advocate, and his intercessor. I wasn't looking to abdicate a whit of responsibility, I explained; in fact, I expected to be continually engaged, actively working to make his next placement work well for everyone involved. Yes, I acknowledged, Dan has behavioral as well as physical challenges—as is typical of severe TBI survivors. But he's a good person worthy of benevolent treatment, dignity, and however much enjoyment he can obtain given the limitations imposed on him by a calamitous accident some four decades earlier.

Shiloh nodded at my summation. The year before, she said, her mother had also survived a TBI—not as severe as Dan's, but serious enough that the issues Dan has faced over the years were all too familiar. I was right, she said: too many people, even professionals in the field of care provision, don't understand and so don't distinguish among developmental deficits, dementia, and TBI. Each is a different condition, presenting different issues that require different strategies and responses. And as far as Shiloh was concerned, Dan's problems as I had described them fit within Harbor Health's purview.

One more thing, I interjected, hoping the stipulation didn't sink us: Dan insisted that he would only move to Indiana if he were allowed to stay in bed. Unclothed. "I think over time he might change his mind," I added, "but I can't know for sure."

Shiloh again nodded. "We would encourage him to get up," she said, "but like everything else at Harbor, the decision would be his. We make suggestions we believe are in our residents' best interest, and we insist on measures to ensure their safety, but they're in charge of their own lives here. Resident choice is our ruling principle."

Perfect.

Barring anything prohibitive in his medical records and paperwork, Shiloh continued, Harbor Health would gladly welcome Dan—and me—in partnership to help him achieve the best life possible for him, on his own terms. She then escorted me through the facility, and the favorable impression developed in her office was only fortified by the tour. The entire building had been recently updated, Shiloh told me, and it seemed to have been designed and appointed with aesthetics as well as function in mind. The color palette had been chosen in accordance with a study on the effects of different colors on mood, and the deep golds, persimmons, and leaf greens of the walls soothed without stultifying. The framed prints were institutionally nondescript but pleasant. Spotless wood-laminate flooring gleamed, both in the hallways and the residents' rooms. In fact, the whole place shone. The rooms seemed a bit smaller than those at Trinity Village but much more cheerful—instead of pocked cement blocks painted a muddy mustardy beige, the walls were unblemished drywall, freshly painted in those serenely uplifting colors, with windows that opened onto a sunny courtyard blooming with geraniums and peonies. The therapy department was well-appointed with an orderly array of specialized machines and gadgets, and near the entrance was Harbor's "Wall of Heroes"—a large bulletin board with the photos and thumbnail success stories of people who had recently benefited from its services. As far as I could see, without exception, the entire facility was attractive, clean, and clearly well organized. And not a whiff of unpleasant odors anywhere—a quality almost impossible to find in a long-term care facility, but critically important in any place I'd want to call home.

By the end of the tour, I knew in my bones that Harbor Health offered what I wanted for Dan. The next step, I realized, was convincing him that, in a world that offered him few acceptable options, this place was an excellent choice, and a choice we could hope for.

★ ★ ★

Dyke and I arranged my four-day visit with Dan little more than a week after my appointment with Shiloh. When I went into Dan's room on Sunday, I held my breath as tightly as I held the laptop that housed my fifty-three-slide PowerPoint argument for Dan moving to Harbor Health. That afternoon, following Dyke's departure for Indiana, I sat beside Dan on his bed and placed my laptop on his chest, already displaying the first slide: planted among well-tended flowers and shrubs, a white sign identifying Harbor Health of Muncie in sweeping dark blue script. I then slowly advanced the slides, reading my titles, elaborating on the significance of each one and offering details, answering whatever questions Dan asked. I had included many snapshots of the facility itself—residents' rooms, nurses' desks, lounge areas, dining rooms, courtyards—that conveyed Harbor's emphasis on aesthetics, cleanliness, and order, augmented by my verbal commentary. ("I swear to you, there aren't any bad smells there. *None*. I'm not kidding.") We went through pictures of the therapy department, illustrating its equipment and its Wall of Heroes, which I hoped might rekindle, in some deep recess, Dan's previously indefatigable aspiration for improvement. ("Shiloh said you don't ever have to get out of bed again, but if you change your mind, you'd be eligible for at least a year of physical therapy.") Dan scrutinized the images, mulling them over. We then scrolled through slides of photos I'd lifted from Harbor's Facebook page, which I'd clustered under the heading OUTINGS AND ACTIVITIES. The VISITING FARM: residents, under a late summer Indiana sky, cradled chicks and patted lambs, calves, and goats. The COMMUNITY EASTER EGG HUNT: clusters of children gathered multicolored plastic eggs sprinkled across a lavishly green expanse of lawn, while residents arrayed in a bank of wheelchairs watched them like proud grandparents or great-grandparents at a Tiny Tots match. MARDI GRAS: residents mugged for the camera in outlandish hats and feathered masks. CASINO DAY: a man studiously worked the lever of a portable slot machine. These images were followed by others I'd labeled AT THE ZOO, FISHING, HUMAN BOARD GAME, THANKSGIVING, and CHRISTMAS. As I moved through these photos, Dan exhibited interest so slight I interpreted it as merely polite. But his attentiveness skyrocketed when we arrived at the series labeled KENTUCKY DERBY DAY. Residents patted ponies in a sunny courtyard. A pair of ponies clopped down one of the polished wooden floor hallways. A pony nuzzled a resident in the dining room. Finally, two snapshots showed a pony nosing a resident in her room. After a running patter of commentary, I fell silent as Dan studied each photo, drinking in the details, and then asked to see them again.

After the second pass, Dan spelled, "HORSE."

"Well, ponies, anyway. I'm not saying they cruise the halls all the time, but apparently it happens sometimes." I paused. "So what do you think? Will you come to Indiana? To Harbor Health? It's entirely your call. But if you decide to move, know that I'll do everything I can to make your life better. I'll be right beside you every step of the way."

The silence that followed felt like minutes as Dan considered his binary options: stay or go. He nodded slowly. "MUNCIE," he spelled.

I put my hand on his and squeezed his fingers. "You'll be glad you made this decision, Dan. As of this moment, we're in it together. I won't let you down, I promise." The calmness of my voice amazed me, because inwardly I was jubilant. But my exuberance was also muted by the gravity of the promise I had just made: "I won't let you down." I pledged to myself in that moment that, in a world that had let Dan down so often, so deeply, and in so many ways, I would absolutely keep it.

★ ★ ★

Later that afternoon, while Dan and I were chatting, a nurse swooped in with a syringe.

"What's that?" I asked.

"Just a little something that helps Dan feel better. Right, Dan?"

He was noncommittal but winced briefly as the nurse briskly poked the needle into his deltoid. Sounds like medication for anxiety, or maybe an anti-depressant, I thought, before thinking no more about it.

★ ★ ★

Because of the enormity of the change I was asking Dan to take on, and especially in light of his compromised abilities (particularly his inability to speak) and how thoroughly his well-being depended on the benevolent care of others, I wasn't surprised when I entered Dan's room the next morning and the first word he spelled was "ATLANTA." After sleeping on the idea, Dan thought he might want to stay at Trinity Village after all. He looked a bit sheepish, because he knew how much I wanted him to relocate.

"It's a big, life-changing decision, and it's absolutely your choice. I want you to be sure of whatever you want to do," I said. "Let's analyze each option through pros and cons and see what makes the most sense to you." I opened up my laptop to take notes. "So what are the pros of staying in Atlanta?" I asked. "What do you like about Trinity Village? What would make you want to stay?"

Dan concentrated thoughtfully, searching for an answer, or perhaps for the word that would encapsulate his answer. After long moments of silence, I offered, "Familiarity?" Enthusiastically, he nodded. I typed Familiarity under Pros. "What else?" I asked.

He thought hard for a time, but neither of us could think of anything. "Let's come back to the Pros in a minute," I said. "What about cons?"

This, apparently, was an easier question. Following his spellings, I typed, Meals are late, cold, and not very tasty. Much of the staff is slow to respond to requests and less than friendly when family isn't around. "And now that Dave is in Maryland, family wouldn't be around as much," I added. He nodded—a definite con.

"What else?" I asked. We came up blank. "I guess since you've started staying in bed and watching TV all the time," I said, "there's not much to say either for or against it. Should we try Muncie now?" We thought a moment. "The situation in Muncie might be even harder to analyze," I mused. "Except for the photos I showed you last night, and what I've told you about my tour and visit with Shiloh, Harbor's one big blank unknown for you. It's my impression that it would be a better place. But, again, since you just plan to lie in bed and watch TV, there's not a lot to go on. Although," I offered, "I can promise you'd be less lonely. I'd be visiting you a lot in Muncie—much more than I can if you're in Atlanta. Dave said he'd visit you with about the same frequency, either place. And Muncie's actually a closer drive for him."

Dan paused a moment, then smiled—if a bit anxiously—and spelled "MUNCIE."

"Muncie it is," I said, smiling back.

★ ★ ★

Family relationships are almost universally important to people, but family has been geometrically more significant for Dan, for whom it has been his most reliable—and, for much of his life, his only—source of social connection. Abundant scholarly research highlights the significance of social connectedness using various terms: belonging, acceptance, connectedness, inclusion; and its opposites: ostracism, rejection, exclusion, bullying; and the ramifications of the absence of connection: isolation, loneliness, alienation. Predominant theorizing points out that our human species is radically social, with the need for sociality rooted in our DNA.[1] We deeply fear exclusion because of inclusion's evolutionary survival value. Humans have always needed each other to survive—to care for each other in youth, old age, infirmity, and sickness; to share food when hunting or foraging hasn't gone well; to help build shelters and to offer refuge during or after a storm; to join in mutual defense when attacked. As a result, the theory goes, we have evolved to experience social distance and relational interruption as existential threats. We fear the absence of social ties because our degree of relatedness can be, in some situations and some contexts, a matter of literal life or death. And just as physical pain is an organism's evolutionarily developed signal to correct a physical threat (we instantly retract our hand from a hot stove, for example), so social isolation results in the pain called loneliness to spur us to action. Loneliness moves us to align our self-presentation and our behavior with societal standards in a bid to restore our standing within the community, or to somehow make amends to repair damaged or disrupted relationships.

As a result, cultural norms help define guidelines to foster (among other things) individuals' social acceptance. When we have transgressed those norms, there are culturally established strategies we can employ to modify our behaviors or negotiate our identities in ways that bring us into the social fold or restore our place within it. For example, we may offer sound reasons for our inability to conform to a given norm or try to shift focus from a standard we can't attain to one we excel in meeting. We may apologize for an aberrant action or behavior and promise to do better in the future, and then dutifully act on that promise. We may try to flatter or charm our way into others' good graces. We may even try to buy our way into acceptance with gifts, material or nonmaterial, or offers of assistance or amusement. Broadly speaking, we attempt to show others that we are reliable, positive partners in sociality who merit inclusion.

But all of these strategies require the ability both to fulfill behavioral expectations and to competently communicate. Consider the plight, then, of a person who is intrinsically unable to establish his social value—who can't reliably conform to behavioral norms, and who can't explain why. Such a person has no constructive way to respond to the social pain of loneliness, no means of effectively, consistently performing actions and behaviors that foster inclusion or restore it when actions or behaviors go awry. And no way to alleviate the pain of loneliness that presses him to span that fearsome gap he can't bridge.

Consider the plight, that is, of Dan, who, when I asked him a few years ago how he would characterize his life since his accident, responded with a single word: "LONELY." In effect and on the whole then, as illuminated by theories of social connection, his answer revealed that for roughly four decades, his life has been typified by existential fear and incessant psychic pain.

★ ★ ★

Even before boarding the flight to Indiana, I emailed Shiloh to give her the good news of Dan's decision to move to Muncie. Before the week was out, with a sheaf of documents Dave UPSed to me in hand, I visited the local LifeStream office to transfer Dan's Medicaid eligibility to Indiana and made a series of phone calls to complete the process. I provided Shiloh with the information Harbor needed to request his records from Trinity Village, a process she said typically took twenty to thirty days.

So the countdown started on August 20, 2017. By mid- to late September, I thought, Dan will be arriving in Muncie. I was excited, but also nervous, experiencing something akin to what I imagine an expectant parent might feel before the birth of her first child: eagerness commingled with an overwhelming sense of responsibility, accompanied by self-doubt and a fear that she won't be up to the task. But I assured myself that I would meet whatever challenges arose, however imperfectly, just as nervous new parents do: fueled by love and guided by an unflagging determination to do my best. Surely my best would be enough. And so I waited, counting the days.

I only counted four, however, before the wait was extended. On August 24, Shiloh emailed me with the news that the medical records she'd received from Trinity Village had raised some questions, and she asked me to call her. When I did, the first thing she said was, "You didn't tell me your brother was schizophrenic."

Assuming I had heard correctly, I wondered if Trinity Village had sent someone else's records. "He's not," I replied, flabbergasted.

"It's in his records," Shiloh said.

"Then there's been some mistake," I answered. "He's never had any symptoms of schizophrenia—no hallucinations, no delusions."

"He's on medication for it—he's on Risperdal."

"I've never heard of that. What is it?"

"An antipsychotic," she said.

My head was swimming. Was that what the nurse had given him during my visit in July—not an anti-anxiety calmative or an anti-depressant but an antipsychotic? I was stunned to silence.

"We'll need more information before we can continue processing Dan's application," Shiloh said. "We need to know when he was diagnosed with schizophrenia, who diagnosed him and on what basis, when he began taking Risperdal, and specifically what condition it was meant to control or eliminate."

Even through my fog, I thought, those are all questions I want answered, too.

But the surprises kept coming. "There's also a notation in his chart that says he was 'unresponsive' one day last month. We need to know who made that determination and exactly what it means."

I told her that I was as surprised as she was by these notes and that I'd get answers for her as soon as I could. That afternoon, I made several calls to Trinity Village to track down whomever I needed to speak to and left urgent voicemails for callbacks as soon as possible. The first call I made, however, was to Dave, who happened to be visiting Dan at Trinity Village that very afternoon. When I told him what was in the records Shiloh had received, he was as shocked and bewildered as I was. Dave had retired from the Navy from a decades-long career as a medical corpsman, so he had an informed understanding of the problems that an antipsychotic, erroneously prescribed, could cause. I became increasingly alarmed as we talked, and we agreed that the Risperdal should be discontinued that very day. Dave relayed our decision to a nurse, who told him that Dan had been receiving the injections for, she guessed, about a year, or whenever he was diagnosed with schizophrenia—a diagnosis never shared with Dan or his family.

The nurse could offer no explanation for Dan's reported unresponsiveness, but Dave had a hunch about what the note might have referred to. Both Dave and I had experienced occasions when Dan simply didn't react at all to questions we'd ask on the phone, even to yes/no prompts that required no more than a vocal interjection. That afternoon Dave asked Dan about it, and Dan acknowledged that at times when he tried to vocalize, he was unable to produce any sound. We now wondered if this problem were related to Risperdal. In fact, in retrospect, we wondered how much of Dan's apparent decline over the past few years might have been attributable to drugs he'd been given. As I reported in an email to Shiloh that evening, "Dan may well need some sort of medication, but he is not schizophrenic . . . and I think it will turn out that Risperdal has been more of a problem than a solution."

★ ★ ★

How and why had Dan been diagnosed with schizophrenia, when he was not schizophrenic? Why was he being injected with an antipsychotic, when he was not psychotic? I was dumbfounded by the revelations in his medical records from Trinity Village. I immediately began researching the issues the records had raised.

I had little specialized training for pursuing complex medical matters. The extent of my medical training was a six-month course I took in 1975 at the Southern California College of Medical and Dental Careers, which equipped me for a brief stint working as a medical assistant for a three-doctor family practice. (I enjoyed the medical field in the abstract, but four months of the day-to-day contact with pain and bodily effluvia was more than I could bear. Still, the basic understanding of anatomy and medical terms I gleaned in that period has proven surprisingly useful over the years.) Decades later, in the process of earning my master's degree and then my PhD, I had become adept at research in my field, but I'd had no formal training for navigating or interpreting the ocean of professional medical knowledge available on the internet. Nevertheless, within the first few hours of exploration, facts and descriptions began falling together into place like puzzle pieces. The picture that was forming was ugly, and downright traumatic.

Before the week was out, I was fairly well-informed about schizophrenia. Everything I learned about this illness reinforced my certainty that Dan had never exhibited any sign of it. My research also unearthed a practice I had never heard of before: chemical restraint. Learning about this practice starkly illuminated Dan's situation. His life at Trinity Village, particularly over the previous few years, took on a new and sinister cast.

The portrait of Trinity Village that formed was one of gross incompetence at best, flagrant malpractice and utter indifference to Dan's well-being at worst.

Schizophrenia, which tends to manifest in late adolescence or early adulthood, involves an imbalance in brain chemistry, specifically of dopamine and glutamate, which convey signals along neural pathways that control perception, thinking, and motivation. This chemical imbalance is characterized by psychosis—an inability to separate imagined phenomena from reality. The classic symptoms of schizophrenia are delusions (false beliefs that persist despite evidence that they are untrue) and hallucinations (seeing or hearing things that aren't actually present). As a result, schizophrenic behavior is often bizarre, as the person responds to hallucinations and filters both real and imaginary stimuli through delusional thinking.

Having known Dan throughout his entire life, through an almost dizzying array of conditions and situations, I could categorically affirm that he had never exhibited the slightest indication of schizophrenia. Despite the extremity of situations he has been forced to deal with since his injury, he has consistently remained thoroughly grounded in external reality. He does exhibit a common TBI-related tendency to disbelieve the severity or permanence of some of his impairments, but that's a disturbance in the way he applies objective information relating to his own physiological state, not an inability to differentiate between real and imagined perceptions.

Risperdal, the drug that Dan had been receiving for at least a year at Trinity Village, is an antipsychotic aimed at correcting the brain chemistry imbalances involved in schizophrenia, bipolar disorder, and autism. Of course, when a chemically balanced brain is subjected to a drug that alters its chemistry, the result is chemical imbalance, which consequently is likely to create mental and physical disequilibrium. Like many drugs, Risperdal carries the risk of side effects—some common, others infrequent, and still others rare. Common side effects are drowsiness, dizziness, agitation and anxiety, and trembling extremities. Infrequently, some of the conditions the drug may cause include low blood pressure, weakness, and confusion. Rarely, the person may experience (among other problems) altered consciousness, falling, joint stiffness, muscle spasms, numbness, difficulty sleeping, urinary tract infections, decreased peristaltic movement, and intestinal blockage.

Schizophrenia is a debilitating illness for those who suffer from it, and most of the side effects that may occur from pharmacological treatment are generally more manageable and less distressing than the effects of the illness itself. Consequently, Risperdal can be positively life-changing for people with schizophrenia, balancing their brain chemistry and helping them to live relatively normal, well-adjusted lives. However, the risks posed by dosing someone without psychosis with this or any other antipsychotic can be severely debilitating, and some of the negative effects may persist weeks or months after discontinuing the drug. In some cases, it can cause permanent damage or even death.

I discovered that in 2013, Janssen Pharmaceuticals (a subdivision of Johnson & Johnson) was convicted of marketing Risperdal to nursing homes as a viable solution to behavioral problems posed by residents, including those who do not suffer from schizophrenia, bipolar disorder, or autism.[2] The antipsychotic's sedative effect reduces unwanted behavior by compromising residents' ability to think, feel, and react to stimuli, often to the point of functionally immobilizing them. Such people are the victims of chemical restraint—the practice of using a drug, or a combination of drugs, to control someone's behavior by incapacitating them, making them easier for nursing home staff to manage.

Chemical restraint is also a matter of law. Administering antipsychotics to nursing home residents who aren't psychotic, debilitating them and putting them at risk for serious mental and physical complications as an answer to behavioral issues unrelated to psychosis, is all too common, but it isn't an authorized practice. As the advocacy organization Human Rights Watch argues, "[C]hemical restraint—for staff convenience or to discipline or punish a resident—could constitute abuse under domestic law and cruel, inhuman, and degrading treatment under international law."[3] The 2013 lawsuit against Janssen Pharmaceuticals placed a spotlight on the issue. And at least in theory, Medicaid and Medicare, the two primary sources of funding for residents in long-term care facilities, approve payment for pharmaceuticals only when they are prescribed according to FDA-endorsed guidelines. The FDA doesn't endorse immobilizing residents with drugs used to treat illnesses they don't have.

Every indication pointed to the conclusion that those in charge of directing Dan's care had been remarkably indifferent to his well-being. The revelations that arose from juxtaposing his medical record with authoritative research sources pointed to utter disregard for his health, safety, and essential humanity. He had been devalued—silenced, immobilized, and endangered—and the degree of betrayal I felt was stunning.

The light had dawned. The only mystery that remained was how Dan had been diagnosed with schizophrenia. Given his aphasia and behavioral issues, indisputably consequences of his TBI, he just as easily (and just as falsely) could have been tagged with bipolar disorder or autism instead.

Notes

1. Roy F. Baumeister and Mark R. Leary, "The Need to Belong: Desire for Interpersonal Attachments as a Fundamental Human Motivation" *Psychological Bulletin* 117, no. 3 (1995): 497–529. doi: 10.1037/0033-2909.117.3.497; Geoff MacDonald and Mark R. Leary, "Why Does Social Exclusion Hurt? The Relationship between Social and Physical Pain" *Psychological Bulletin* 131, no. 2 (2005): 202–23. doi: 10.1037/0033-2909.131.2.202; John T. Cacioppo and William Patrick, *Loneliness: Human Nature and the Need for Social Connection* (New York: W.W. Norton & Company, 2008); Kipling D. Williams, Joseph P. Forgas, and William von Hippel, *The Social Outcast: Ostracism, Social Exclusion, Rejection, and Bullying* (New York: Psychology Press, 2014); and Kelly-Ann Allen, *The Psychology of Belonging* (London: Routledge, Taylor & Francis Group, 2021).
2. Eric Holder, *Attorney General Press Conference Transcript*. www.justice.gov/opa/speech/attorney-general-eric-holder-delivers-remarks-johnson-johnson-press-conference, November 4, 2013.
3. Hannah Flamm, *"They Want Docile": How Nursing Homes in the United States Overmedicate People with Dementia* (New York: Human Rights Watch, 2018), 2.

2 Correcting the Record

After two weeks of my urgent phone calls to Trinity Village and countless voicemails I left scattered through its various offices, Shiloh finally received some additional medical records for Dan but no official answers to the fundamental questions she was asking: what was the basis of Dan's schizophrenia diagnosis, who had prescribed the Risperdal, and precisely when had he begun receiving the drug? Without acceptable answers to those questions, she said, Harbor Health would not accept Dan as a resident. Shiloh's concern for the safety of staff and other residents necessitated documented assurance that he wasn't violent. Since Harbor had no dedicated "behavioral wing" (read: psychiatric unit) to place him into until a professional evaluation could be made, she sent me contact information for another Muncie nursing home, with the suggestion that Dan might temporarily transfer there to undergo a psychiatric assessment. Once he'd been cleared of disqualifying issues, we could renew his application to Harbor.

Knowing that getting Dan to agree to that plan of action was unlikely, and unwilling to put him through the stress of it anyway, I decided to press Trinity Village to perform the reassessment. It was only fair; a new evaluation was only necessary because their records contained gaps and a false diagnosis. At the same time, I thought it prudent to begin a search for an acceptable alternative to Harbor—a decent facility in the area that might take Dan even with the inaccuracies in his record—in case correcting his records took too long. Now that Dave was in Maryland, I was keenly aware of how alone Dan felt by himself in Georgia. Additionally, I was anxious to get him out of Trinity Village. In truth, I had lost all confidence in the place where he had been misdiagnosed and, until just weeks before, chemically restrained.

The next day, Shiloh emailed me scans of the most recent records Trinity Village had sent her. I was dumbfounded to discover that, in addition to the misdiagnosis of schizophrenia, Trinity Village had somehow

DOI: 10.4324/9781003340294-2

determined that Dan was also afflicted with schizoaffective disorder, anxiety disorder, major depressive disorder, and cerebral palsy, in addition to the TBI he actually (and only) did have.

I could hardly catch my breath. All of these diagnoses were now part of Dan's medical record, which would accompany his application to any facility I tried to bring him into. On the basis of Trinity Village's records, what kind of "home" would Dan be considered fit for? What would I be able to offer him? Not likely one with brightly lit hallways, gleaming wood-laminate flooring, and walls freshly painted in colors both cheerful and serene; or one with a Wall of Heroes honored by its therapy department; or one that offered bedridden residents the chance to nuzzle ponies. How was I going to keep the promise I'd made?

One evening later that week, I dropped in on the nursing home Shiloh had recommended. I came away crushed. It wasn't hellish, but it wasn't far from purgatory, either. It struck me as dismal—no place I wanted Dan to stay, even temporarily. The building was old, with the same Trinity Village-beige-cinderblock walls. The hallways were gloomy, lit by dim, flickering fluorescent lights. The staff was indifferent, hardly noticing and not at all marking my presence, and the air was subtly tainted with the odor of excreta. As it turned out, my negative impression was irrelevant. When I called the director the next day, I discovered that, while the facility was in the final stage of adding an Alzheimer's unit, it didn't have a behavioral wing or conduct psychiatric evaluations. Even if I had wanted to bring Dan into the place, which I didn't, it wouldn't have accepted him.

Having so thoroughly sold Dan on Harbor and conjuring up visions of the bright new life awaiting him in Muncie, I couldn't begin to imagine how I would break the news.

★ ★ ★

Uncertain that Harbor would eventually accept Dan, and with online research and spontaneous visits to other local nursing homes casting doubt that acceptable (and accepting) alternatives to Harbor existed in Muncie, my search for a place for Dan expanded. Dorrie, a family friend, was the director of housekeeping at The Haven, a nursing home in a small town just beyond the outskirts of Muncie, and she offered to give Dyke and me a tour of the facility. The Haven would add another twenty-five minutes of driving time each way to visits—inconvenient, certainly, but well worth the extra time and gas if Plan A (Harbor) fell through. When I told Dorrie that Dan had been chemically restrained at Trinity Village, she was incensed. That would never happen at *her* facility, she fumed. I was ready to be favorably impressed.

Dyke and I drove out to The Haven on a Sunday afternoon in mid-September. The facility shimmered in the warm golden sunlight of early fall, set within a thick semicircle of trees just beginning to infuse their green leaves with lemony yellow.

The brick building was about the same age as Harbor's, but the interior lacked Harbor's remodeled, updated feel. Nevertheless, it was clearly well maintained, the staff Dorrie introduced us to were friendly and earnest, and the air was pleasant in every corner. I was more than satisfied with its cleanliness and homey feel. Harbor was still my first choice, but if that possibility fell through, I believed Dan would be in good hands at The Haven.

The following week, I emailed Dan's records to The Haven's administrator with a note intended to defuse their negative portrait of my brother, proactively offering a more positive, yet conscientiously truthful, one. I began,

> I'm acutely aware of the view of Dan that any reasonable person might draw from his medical records. To add another voice, I'm including in this email some background from the perspective of his family. I realize it is somewhat long, but I do believe it draws a truer, more balanced picture of Dan and his situation.

I then recounted what I had told Shiloh in her office, explaining the necessity of moving Dan so that family was nearby, and describing his physical and behavioral difficulties. I included the 2012 Trinity Village accusation that he had attacked a staff member, which I followed with the statement, "I've never seen him actually try to hurt anyone, and to the best of my knowledge, he never has." I countered the misdiagnoses that were charted in his medical records. I explained that at least some of the references to "refused treatment" marked in his chart were either rationally justified in that the proposed "treatment" caused him considerable pain, or were the result of a physical inability to comply with advice he gladly would have followed, if only he were able to. I concluded with the pledge I'd made to Shiloh:

> Wherever Dan ends up, I am going to be very involved in his life. I will be visiting him weekly, phoning him daily, and making myself available as needed (within work constraints). I'm committed to staying close both to my brother and to facility staff, to help in any way I can. I understand that my responsibility doesn't end when he is admitted into a facility, nor do I want it to. I'm a very willing partner in the effort to restore some quality—to whatever degree restoration is possible—to my brother's life.

In reply, the administrator thanked me for my "perspective" and noted that the nursing notes were missing for June, July, and September. She asked me to contact Trinity Village with a request to send records that filled that gap. When I made the request, the social worker at Trinity Village informed me that since Dan wasn't on their skilled nursing program, and there hadn't been any additional procedures or events to log over those periods, there were no entries to provide. I sent The Haven's administrator the social worker's phone number so that she could contact her directly, but I don't know whether or not she ever did. Within weeks, when I realized I couldn't obtain the information The Haven wanted in a timely manner, I asked that Dan's application be placed on hold until I could supply the missing documentation (although I had no idea how I would fulfill that assignment). My request was proactive. Clearly, I was going to need more time to prevent another rejection.

★ ★ ★

Between teaching classes and grading papers, September passed in a flurry of phone calls and emails as I tried to arrange a psychiatric reassessment for Dan at Trinity Village. On October 3, which was just over two weeks past the time he would have been scheduled to receive his next Risperdal injection, I entered in my journal, "Tonight, for the first time in a very long time, he told me 'BYE' before we hung up. So he seems to be coming back around a bit, which gives me hope." To explain the delay in bringing him to Indiana without angering or alarming him by specifics while remaining truthful, I told him that errors in his medical record had caused difficulties in getting the paperwork through with Harbor. I assured him—with a confidence I didn't entirely possess—that I would get it worked out. I was certainly trying.

I had an appointment for a phone meeting with Paula Owens, Trinity Village's Director of Health Services. The previous week, I'd had an unpleasant and unproductive conversation with Dan's assigned social worker at the facility that, by the end of the call, bordered on acrimony from both sides. So I prepared for my conversation with Paula by organizing an outline to help me stay calm and on target. During our meeting, I took careful notes by fleshing out my outline, and this call went much better.

Despite the hard-boiling anger I felt following the revelation that Trinity Village had been subjecting Dan to chemical restraint, I wanted to start my conversation with Paula on a positive note, so I began somewhat disingenuously by telling her that Dave and I appreciated the care our brother had received at her facility for the previous eleven years. I didn't mention that the quality of his care dropped significantly after Trinity

Village was acquired by a large conglomerate in 2009, or that the status quo dipped several notches further in 2013, after Dan had been accused of trying to "run down" a staff member. And I certainly didn't mention the term *chemical restraint*. Instead, I began by simply accentuating the positive: Dan's family appreciated that Trinity Village had been providing his care for such a long time.

We wanted to move Dan, I said, not because of anything Trinity Village had done or not done—which was true; when I began the process of trying to transfer Dan to Indiana, I had no idea that he was being immobilized with an antipsychotic. I felt no need to inform Paula of my self-education regarding chemical restraint or my conviction that Trinity Village had pharmaceutically abused my brother. Instead, I explained that we wanted Dan to move to Indiana because Dave had left Georgia for Maryland in July, and it was important for Dan to live near family. Paula echoed the point that being near family was critical to residents' well-being. I noted that I had scheduled this phone meeting with Paula because I had been stymied by an unexpected snag: when the Indiana facility we had chosen received Dan's medical records from Trinity Village, his application had been at least temporarily rejected due to some mysterious entries in his chart. I hoped to get clarification from Paula for what I didn't understand and to obtain corrections for what I knew to be inaccuracies in Dan's records.

Paula expressed surprise at my mention of inaccuracies, and I studiously tried to avoid the slightest whiff of accusation. "I just don't believe his record gives an accurate picture of who Dan is," I told her. "Because he's aphasic, he's not been able to explain his thoughts or elaborate on his reasons for various actions, and I believe that, as a result, some misleading conclusions were drawn." I explained that I was not asking for—and indeed, didn't want—anything untrue to be placed in his record or anything true to be removed; I merely hoped to offer some of what I knew about my brother so that the record could more accurately reflect who Dan is and what his next facility should reasonably expect—including the challenges he posed. With what was currently in his medical record, I told her, Dan was likely to be accepted only by a psychiatric facility, which was not where he belonged. Paula agreed with satisfying alacrity that he didn't belong in a psychiatric unit, and I was genuinely thankful for that. I emphasized that I didn't want to soft-pedal his difficulties; I simply wanted a true, more complete picture of who Dan is and what he's like.

What, Paula asked, did I consider inaccurate? The most serious problem, I said, was the roster of diagnoses listed for Dan: schizophrenia, schizoaffective disorder, anxiety disorder, and major depressive disorder. How, I asked, were these diagnoses obtained? Dan is aphasic, I noted, but he has never suffered from delusions or hallucinations, the hallmarks of schizophrenia. Who had decided he had these illnesses, and on what evidence? What had Dan conveyed in interviews, or what tests had been done, and by whom? If these diagnoses had been made during his weeklong observation at Cornerstone Hospital in 2012, I reasoned, consider the conditions surrounding his examination: he'd just been transferred to a mental hospital with no indication of how long he'd be staying there; he was under threat of being evicted from the place he'd lived for the previous six years, with nowhere else to go; and he was unable to speak for himself—powerless to provide details or to convey his perspective about anything he was asked, not to mention his inability to present his side of the incident involving the staff member that had landed him at Cornerstone in the first place. I noted that feeling anxious and depressed (to whatever degree he was able to express those or any other feelings in an interview with someone who didn't know him well and who likely couldn't read fingerspelling anyway) would be an entirely normal reaction to the situation in which he found himself. Paula readily agreed.

Furthermore, I pointed out, there was the baffling diagnosis of cerebral palsy. People are *born* with cerebral palsy, and it manifests by early childhood at the latest. Dan was, by any measurable standard, completely normal until his accident at eighteen years old. He had a traumatic brain injury, not cerebral palsy. Paula expressed her own surprise that such a diagnosis was listed in his chart; *of course* he didn't have cerebral palsy, she said.

I explained that in the wake of these misdiagnoses and my insistence that they were mistaken, our chosen long-term care facility in Muncie had asked for a psychiatric reassessment, and I was hoping that that Trinity Village would arrange it. However, I wanted to be present with Dan and the evaluator so that I could relate Dan's responses to questions, so that his perspective would be given due consideration—a precaution that might have prevented the misdiagnoses in the first place.

Additionally, I said, I hoped for clarification and elaboration on the claim appearing in his records that Dan was "running staff in his motor scooter." What, exactly, did that phrase mean—was he rampaging through the hallways trying to mow down personnel? If so, how many times had this happened? Had he ever collided with, or in any other way injured, anybody? If not, what had stopped him? If he was actually dangerous— violent—what actions had anyone been forced to take in order to prevent him from causing harm to others?

There was the incident in 2012, Paula said, when he had "threatened" someone with his wheelchair, accidentally knocking a cooler of ice off a table. Paula didn't consider him violent, although some of his behavior—occasionally hollering and waving his middle finger at staff—was inappropriate and could even be considered aggressive.

"Inappropriate, yes—but dangerous?" I asked. "Has he ever actually hurt anyone?"

"No," she answered, "but I'm not sure he hasn't tried."

"If he's tried, what's kept him from succeeding?" I asked.

"I don't know."

"Well, if he's going to be labeled as dangerous even though he's never harmed anyone, doesn't the basis of that judgment need to be clarified?"

Yes, she agreed, it does.

I acknowledged that, while Dan doesn't have schizophrenia, or schizoaffective disorder, or anxiety disorder, he does have TBI, which includes the sporadic angry outbursts that are so typically symptomatic of severe brain injury. While admittedly very unpleasant and even disturbing, the episodes pass within a few seconds or minutes, although others can respond in ways that prolong and even intensify them. Paula concurred—Dan's outbursts are unnerving, she said, but they don't seem to present any danger, either to himself or to others.

Next, I noted the repeated appearance in his chart of the word "refusal" in terms of treatment. "I know of at least two instances where he has had good reasons for not doing as he's told, which I suspect is the real problem here," I said. First, when he was advised to shift his weight while lying in bed in order to prevent pressure sores, he hadn't *refused* to comply; he was *unable* to turn himself, and when I tried to help him, he winced in pain. Similarly, in April, his chart said that he had begun "refusing" to get out of bed. I confessed that I hadn't learned until several months later that getting up had been causing him pain, and that was why he had decided to stay in bed. Far from displaying resistance to treatment, I noted, Dan's decision to stay in bed struck me as perfectly reasonable; nobody voluntarily does things that cause them pain. Again, Paula readily agreed.

Our meeting ended with Paula saying that she thought my request for a psychiatric re-evaluation was entirely reasonable. She promised that, while she didn't have Dan's records before her, she would track them down, review them, and get back to me. Unfortunately, she would be on vacation the following week, but she would attend to these issues when she returned to work. I wished her a good vacation, we exchanged a bit of friendly small talk, and then we hung up.

I was elated. Finally! After a month of calls and frequently unanswered voicemails, after repeatedly being handed from one person to another, I had found someone at Trinity Village who understood Dan's plight, who agreed that he didn't belong in a psychiatric ward and so had pledged to arrange a psychological reassessment that I could be present for—in brief,

I had found an ally at Trinity Village who was in a position to enable Dan's relocation to a good facility near his sister, and who wanted to help make it happen.

But my elation was short-lived. Over the next month, a rash of voicemails I left for Paula went unanswered. When she called me back a month later, it was to tell me that Trinity Village's "psychology team" had visited Dan that very afternoon, and she would send me a copy of the resultant report as soon as she received it. She explained that the team would likely follow up with Dan in a few weeks, and she'd try to give me advance notice of the date for Dan's reassessment so that I could arrange to be present.

During a visit with Dan a few days later, when I asked him how his meeting with the psychology team had gone, he looked at me quizzically. After a moment's thought, he told me that a stranger had briefly entered his room—for "THIRTY SECONDS" or so—but she didn't introduce herself, and he had no idea why she was there. He thought maybe she had walked into the wrong room. She was gone so swiftly, and it had seemed such a nonevent, that he hadn't given it another thought.

At this point, it had been three months since Dan had agreed to move to Indiana, and four months since Dave had left Georgia. After another two weeks, when there was no more word from Paula and no more mention of a psychology team, a report, or a scheduled reassessment, I decided to bypass Trinity Village entirely. On November 16, I emailed the Georgia State Governor's Office of Disability Services Ombudsman. My message read, in part,

> I have been trying to resolve this issue by working with staff at Trinity Village. The Health Services Director agreed in October that a re-evaluation is in order to correct Dan's record. She seems willing to help, but there have been no real signs of progress in the six weeks since we first discussed the issue. In the meantime, Dan has been feeling increasingly isolated and frustrated for reasons that are both unfair and beyond his (or my) control. All I want is to move the re-evaluation process forward so that I can successfully make the arrangements necessary to bring Dan to live near me.
>
> Can your office help us?

In less than a week, the Ombudsman's office contacted me with the news that Trinity Village had scheduled Dan's psychological reassessment for December 4—two weeks later. By the time I received the news, however, there was a real question whether or not Dan would live long enough to keep the appointment.

★ ★ ★

The call from Trinity Village came just after midnight on Monday, November 21. Dan had been transported to the emergency room at nearby Sugarbush Hospital. Nobody knew exactly what was wrong with him, but he was in serious danger. After repeated calls to the hospital, and even though I was one of the two people on Dan's list of family members, due to HIPA (privacy laws) the only information the hospital would release to me was that he was indeed in the emergency room. I faced a long, sleepless night in Indiana, 600 miles away from my brother. I keenly felt every mile.

I got a fuller story the next morning from Dave, who had just visited Dan on Saturday. When I called Dan Saturday morning, he was looking forward to a rousing afternoon of pizza and football, which Dave told me had gone well; they'd had a great time together, as usual, and Dan was upbeat, quick to laugh at Dave's jokes. Dave spent the next day with his son Chris and his family, who lived in the area. He called Dan several times but got no answer, which was highly unusual, but since Trinity Village hadn't called to report any problems, Dave didn't think more about it.

When Dave went to Trinity Village on Monday morning before returning to Maryland, however, he was shocked by Dan's appearance. He later told me, "It looked like he'd be dead within a few hours." (Because of Dave's twenty-some years as a Navy corpsman, he knows what impending death looks like.) Later I would learn that, earlier that morning when the nursing staff changed shifts at 7:00 a.m., Dan's roommate Frank insistently ushered Addie, a certified nursing assistant (CNA), to Dan's bedside. "Dan was in a terrible state," she told me. His eyes were sunken, his skin was flaccid, and he was in obvious pain. Addie sat with Dan all morning and afternoon, spooning ice chips into his mouth to combat dehydration. She contacted the nurse practitioner on duty, who ordered IV fluids, blood work, and a chest x-ray. Within a few hours, the x-ray results returned as normal, but when the lab results came back that night, the ambulance was summoned to take Dan to the emergency room.

By the time I spoke with Dave on Tuesday morning, Dan had been diagnosed with sepsis, a systemic chemical imbalance triggered by an infection that sent his body's immune response into toxic overdrive. I knew just how serious that condition could be, as Dyke's aunt had died from it a few years earlier. Dave didn't try to downplay the danger, opting instead to prepare me: "Katie, he might not make it." An IV drip was flooding Dan's body with high-powered antibiotics, with the aim of bringing the infection under control before his organs began shutting down. He was already in renal crisis, and his blood pressure was dangerously low. His abdomen was greatly distended, and a CT scan revealed a shadow around his gall bladder, suggestive of gall stones or a tumor, which could be cancerous. In short, he was on the threshold of death, and while he was receiving intense, expert care, doctors couldn't yet say on which side of the threshold he'd land.

Later that afternoon, Dave reported that Dan was more alert and seemed to be doing a bit better. He had been moved from Intensive Care to the Intermediate Care Unit, which Dave found highly encouraging. In his experience, when people died of sepsis, he said, "once it kicks in, they only spiral down." So Dan's signs of improvement, however small, were hopeful. Dan, Dave, and Dan's doctor, Dr. Khan, had met in Dan's room a few hours earlier. To resolve the mystery presented by the shadow around his gall bladder, Dr. Khan noted that surgery was a possibility, but she was hesitant to undertake it. In addition to sepsis, tests revealed that Dan was seriously dehydrated and malnourished. Dr. Khan feared that, in his weakened state, he might not survive an operation. Together, the three of them tabled the idea of surgery for the moment, reserving it as a strategy of last resort.

The news that Dan was malnourished was shocking. It was hard to fathom how I could have failed to notice on our visits how thin he had become. It seemed even stranger that Trinity Village staff had. After all, they bathed him. They brought his meals and took away his trays, still bearing whatever food he hadn't eaten. Had no one seen that he was too thin and that he wasn't eating enough to stay healthy? Weren't they supposed to keep track of such things?

Dave further informed me that, following a candid discussion with Dr. Khan, Dan signed a DNR (Do Not Resuscitate) form. I found this news shocking, too. Admittedly, the drive for self-preservation is instinctive for us all, but Dan's passionate determination to combat all threats, to defy all odds, was a blazing hallmark of his character. This decision indicated not only the extremity he was now facing, but also his weakening resolve to fight it. I didn't blame him; in his place, I would have made the same decision—but resignation comes more easily to me than to my brother.

That night, Dan's nurse gave me a full update and allowed me to ask questions, which she answered without reserve. She noted that Dan's blood pressure was concerningly low, but she was working to raise it. I was allowed to talk to him on the phone for a few minutes, which was a huge boon to my spirits. He was cheerful, and his voice was strong and vigorous, even though I knew he was not.

Sometime after midnight, Dave received a phone call from a doctor seeking approval to put Dan on a pressor, a drug aimed at increasing his blood pressure. The medication was so potent that it would require Dan's transfer back to Intensive Care for observation. Giving Dan the drug was risky, but the doctor felt that not giving it to him would be riskier. Dave made the call to allow the drug. But when he arrived at the hospital the next morning, he learned that Dan's blood pressure had raised sufficiently on its own so that the pressor hadn't been needed. By that evening, his lactic acid level was normal, and his white blood cell count was nearly so. They had removed his nasogastric tube—a tube threaded through his nose, down his esophagus, and into his stomach—and he had taken some liquids by mouth throughout the day: Italian lemon ice, broth, and jello. My journal entry for 10:30 that night reads, "Dan's resting comfortably, isn't in pain, his BP is up to acceptable levels, he's sleeping now but was watching TV and channel surfing. Sounds really positive. Whew! I'll sleep well tonight!"

Dan was in the hospital for the rest of the week and the weekend. His final diagnosis was toxic megacolon that had presented with sepsis. A bit of online research helped me understand the condition that had nearly killed him. Resulting from severe inflammation of the smooth-muscle layers of the colon, toxic megacolon is characterized by severe pain, fever, tachycardia (rapid heartbeat), and hypotension (low blood pressure), a complex of symptoms that signals systemic toxicity. It is, indeed, potentially lethal.

One form of toxic megacolon is idiopathic, or acquired, when it is caused by chronic constipation. Some of the common causes of chronic constipation are a lack of dietary fiber (too few unprocessed foods, especially fruit, vegetables, and whole grains), an insufficient intake of liquids, and a lack of exercise. The discovery that Dan was seriously malnourished was surprising because of the neglect it suggested, but his dysphagia (difficulty swallowing due to oral paralysis) complicated the issue because it does make his eating more difficult. He has struggled with bouts of dehydration for the same reason. And since he had stopped getting out of bed seven months earlier, his activity level had dramatically decreased. All of these circumstances created conditions for a perfect storm leading to chronic constipation. The shadow surrounding Dan's gall bladder turned out to be stool, stalled in his colon because of his loss of peristaltic action.

Since Dan no longer left his bed, every instance of urinating and moving his bowels would have been known to his Trinity Village care providers. They apparently didn't notice or track his increased difficulty with elimination, any more than they had noted his wasting away or his largely uneaten meals.

Another interesting piece of information: within half an hour online, I discovered a suspected, if rare, correlation between toxic megacolon and Risperdal.[1]

Dr. Khan released Dan from the hospital with the recommendation that he enter hospice. Instead, he returned to his old room at Trinity Village. And the urgency I felt to get him out of that place and into a nursing home near me geometrically intensified.

Note

1. Dominic K. Lim and Rathi Mahendran, "Risperidone and Megacolon" *Singapore Medical Journal* 43, no. 10 (October 2002): 530–32; and "Megacolon: What Is It, Causes, Symptoms, Treatment, and More" *Osmosis from Elsevier.* www.osmosis.org/megacolon

3 Dan's Life
1960–1984

Following Dan's near-death hospitalization, I questioned how he had arrived at a state of such extremity in a facility whose mission was ensuring the well-being of people like Dan. Instead of helping him pursue a life worth living, with dignity and the subtle pleasures that come with social integration and engagement, he had been left lying in bed staring at the ceiling, mind fuzzed by drugs, powerless even to adequately conduct the most essential activities of daily life—eating, drinking, and excreting—and unable to communicate his plight. Trinity Village's efforts to eliminate Dan's rage episodes had almost eliminated Dan.

This revelation was appalling, and I was nonplussed. I knew for a fact that Trinity Village was staffed by human beings, not monsters. I didn't know any of the staff well, but I was adequately acquainted with enough of them to know that at least some were well-intentioned. Like Addie, the nurse who sat with Dan all day and spooned ice chips into his mouth to keep him hydrated before he was rushed to the hospital. In light of that kind of compassion, how could Dan have been treated so badly, immobilized with drugs and neglected? What could explain an indifference to his well-being so deep that in effect it had erased him, and in fact had nearly killed him?

It seemed—and to me, this is key—that Dan's treatment at Trinity Village illustrates a claim made by social psychologists: belonging can be a matter of life and death. To be socially valued, recognized by others as one of their own, matters to us on a primal level. The psychosocial stakes of belongingness—one's perception of belonging within the community—are high because of the critical role that others necessarily play in our survival. We are, because we have evolved to be, a radically social species, as a lack of belonging threatens our physical well-being as surely as a lack of food or water. And although the timeline posed by the threat of social deprivation may be longer, the deficiency can be just as lethal.[1]

(It is worth noting that Addie's atypical regard for Dan demonstrates that belonging need not be total in order to be insufficient. It also illustrates the life-and-death nature of belonging, in that Dan likely would not have survived without his roommate Frank's concern and Addie's ice chips.)

In essence, Dan had been insufficiently valued by staff at Trinity Village, denied an overall state of belonging within the community in which he lived. But a lack of belonging had plagued him to varying degrees long before Trinity Village. From the moment Dan regained awareness after his accident and began to grasp the gravity of his situation, he began struggling to regain his status as an esteemed, integral member of society. Like so many (all?) in his situation, every hope, every action, was aimed—directly or indirectly—at restoring a sense of social equilibrium. The events of Dan's postaccident life demonstrate more than the physical hardships that TBI has imposed on him. They also testify both to his efforts to restore an adequate measure of belonging and to the consequences of his inability to secure it.

★ ★ ★

Dan has been living with serious impairments since November of 1978, when he was eighteen years old. He'd been living on a ranch in Oklahoma for three months, working as an apprentice horse trainer while finishing his senior year of high school. Teaching quarter horses to race was demanding, physically and mentally, and he loved it. Horses had been his passion since the day he discovered horseback riding as a fourteen-year-old boy. In the intervening four years, he'd spent most of his spare time working as a groom, first at Carbon Canyon Stables and then at Los Alamitos Race Course near our home in Fullerton, California. Despite his obsession with horses, Dan found time to get good grades in school and to pal around with his best friend Henry, occasionally spending time at the family cabin in the San Bernardino Mountains and learning to water ski on Lake Arrowhead. Early on, he had hoped to become a jockey, but he soon literally outgrew his goal, and his aspirations turned to training young quarter horses to race. Through his job at Los Alamitos he met trainer Will Swift, and it was at Will's ranch outside of Chelsea, Oklahoma, that he intended to finish his senior year of high school while jump-starting his training career as Will's apprentice. At Chelsea High School he began pursuing an additional interest—namely Allie, a bright junior with luminous eyes and an exuberant smile. She and Dan often double-dated with Allie's sister Jane and Dan's new best friend Chuck. The girls were teaching Dan the social arts of line-dancing and two-stepping, but it was Allie who was usually on his arm, boots stomping toward his first real romance.

No one knows why or how it happened, but on November 27, 1978, just after Thanksgiving, Dan was kicked by a horse. Had that horse's hoof struck his head with slightly more force, or at a slightly different angle, or had the ambulance arrived ten minutes later than it did, he might not have survived. My parents, Dave, and I converged in the Tulsa airport from our various locations just after sunrise the next morning. The shock I'd been slogging through since receiving the news of Dan's injury intensified at the airport when my mother collapsed, weeping, into my arms. She was not a weeper.

For the ten weeks Dan remained in Tulsa's St. Francis Hospital, my parents rented one of several studio apartments that the hospital made available to patients' families. Dave and I stayed in the apartment with them for the first two weeks, until Dave's leave from the Navy and my vacation time from work had expired. (I had applied and interviewed for a job at St. Francis in a last-ditch effort at staying with Dan in Tulsa. The interviewer kindly, and wisely, turned me down. It hadn't occurred to me to question what I would have done when Dan left St. Francis and Tulsa.) Eight weeks later, still in a coma but showing the first stirrings of consciousness, Dan was transported by air ambulance to St. Jude's Hospital near our family home in Fullerton. My parents returned from Tulsa with him, and Dan began the long process of regaining as much as possible of what he had lost with the accident: his ability to independently eat, walk, bathe, brush his teeth, comb his hair, shave, button his shirt, tie his shoes, and the myriad other functions most of us take for granted. It was a full-time job, which Dan undertook with the indefatigable presence and persistence that still defined him. And yet, given the sweeping severity of his brain injury, it seemed little short of a miracle when, by July, he was again able to conduct most of the tasks of daily living unassisted, if painstakingly slowly, and was released from St. Jude's. He moved back into the family home, continuing his rehabilitation as an outpatient and studying with a tutor in an attempt to recover his reading and math skills.

★ ★ ★

Dan describes his childhood as generally happy. He has few concrete memories that date back to Miami, where he was born, and not many more of Millen, Georgia, the small rural community we relocated to when he was six years old. A shy boy who didn't make friends easily, his more vivid recollections begin with his friendship with Rocky, his first best friend. Rocky lived in our neighborhood in Statesboro, a small college town in Georgia, where we moved when Dan was nine. Decades later I was surprised to learn from Dan what a hellion Rocky had been—an inveterate shoplifter who stole liquor from his parents' cabinet while he was still prepubescent—because both he and Dan were always so quiet, so apparently well-behaved. Dan was flirting with mischief; he himself didn't participate in the shoplifting, but he accompanied Rocky on the expeditions and vicariously enjoyed the excitement. He did share Rocky's liquor once, when he was ten or eleven; he was sick for two days and resumed his status as spectator, enjoying Rocky's company but declining his friend's encouragement to join in on the delinquency.

When Dan was thirteen, our family relocated again, this time to Fullerton, California. It was a difficult transition. The family was temporarily splintered: Dad remained in Statesboro for a few months in order to sell the house; Dave, seven years older than Dan, stayed behind in Georgia; and I had just started my first year of college at UCLA and was living on campus; so Dan and Mom made the move by themselves. Mom didn't welcome the change; she missed the friends and job she'd left behind, and she plunged into depression. Dan felt utterly lost; he was a stranger at his new school, his father and siblings were absent, his mother was miserable, and Fullerton—a bustling satellite in the Los Angeles area—was an overwhelming change from the comparatively sleepy Southern town we'd left. But after a few months he began settling in. Dad joined Mom and Dan by Christmas, Dave followed soon thereafter, and Dan became friends with Henry, who would remain his best friend until Dan's move to Oklahoma five years later.

The following summer, when he was fourteen, Dan discovered horses at Carbon Canyon Stables. He learned quickly and became an avid rider, and within months Robbie, the manager, hired him as a stable hand. The pay was low—$30 a week—but the benefits were just what Dan was looking for: informal riding instruction, a warm friendship with Robbie, and all the time he could spare spent with horses. He saved his money and bought Dusty, a good-tempered, well-mannered palomino. Together, they won ribbons in local equestrian shows.

Dan began accompanying Robbie and Leon, Carbon Canyon's owner, to Los Alamitos Race Course. Before long, he was working there as a groom, making a cool $100 a week. It was through his work at Los Alamitos that he met Will Swift, who was impressed with Dan's willingness to work hard and cheerfully over long hours for little money. The summer Dan was eighteen, Will hired him as a temporary assistant; they trained horses together on a ranch near Tucson, a project which lasted two months. On their way back to Los Alamitos, Will asked Dan if he'd be interested in working as an apprentice trainer on Will's ranch in Chelsea, Oklahoma, where he could finish his last four months of high school. Dan was delighted to accept the job.

It may seem strange that our parents allowed their teenaged son to make such major decisions as accepting employment at a racetrack and moving several states away to work while he was still in school. But Dan openly discussed his goals and intentions with them, and they never doubted the soundness of his judgment. He was extremely independent, but he was neither rebellious nor delinquent; he was a good-humored, responsible young man who maintained good grades, worked with gusto, saved his money, and had firm educational and vocational goals. Unlike their other two children, Dave and me, Dan had managed to travel through adolescence without any major scrapes or mishaps. They attributed the difference at least in part to Dan's steadfast involvement with horses. That involvement had sailed him safely through a healthy adolescence, and it seemed to have set his course for adulthood. They couldn't have foreseen that in November of 1978, just three months into his life in Chelsea, his pursuit of that course would capsize him.

★ ★ ★

Following Dan's devastating fall at Troy High School in October of 1979, eleven months after his initial TBI, surgeons at St. Jude's replaced his shattered cranial plate. Although he had lost some of the gains he'd made in the hospital's rehabilitation program—and substantial additional ground as well—within a month, Dan was back at Troy. He finished his courses by spring, but he was dissatisfied, feeling that the tutors assigned to help him had completed more of his assigned work than he had, rather than helping him relearn what he needed in order to do the work himself. Dan hadn't entered the program to slide through it; he had a high school diploma, so he didn't need the paper, and he had no use for a certificate that claimed he had skills he still lacked. His aim was to restore what he had lost. So he took a new tack: he enrolled in math and English classes at nearby Santa Ana Community College beginning the following fall.

Over the intervening summer, however, Dan was anything but idle. Along with other forms of therapy, he intensively trained on a driving simulator at St. Jude's rehabilitation center, took private lessons from a driving instructor, and adapted his Toyota pick-up with special devices to compensate for his limited mobility. Before the end of the summer, he had passed the necessary tests and obtained a new California driver's license, an accomplishment of personal significance that could hardly be overstated. Being able to drive again was a tremendous step toward a restored sense of himself as a self-reliant young man moving through the world. He was thrilled that he could drive himself to classes in Santa Ana and to weekly sessions at the Orange County Riding Academy, where straddling a horse again provided both functional physical therapy and the chance to indulge his elemental connection to horses. But above all, driving was a crucial marker of independence and adulthood for him. He was, after all, twenty years old.

Dan had hoped the English class at Santa Ana would help him regain proficiency in reading and writing, but keeping up with the class required capabilities that he lacked. Somehow he had managed to pass the placement test needed to enter the class, so when he failed to complete assignments, the instructor believed he was lazy and indifferent when, in fact, she probably had never had as diligent or motivated a student as Dan. Since he was unable to explain his situation, Mom drove to the campus and told the astonished instructor that Dan was unable to read, and he withdrew from the class. He did complete the math course, however. It took him two semesters to remaster the necessary skills, but he persisted and met his goal.

In 1982, Dad's work situation took Mom, Dad, and Dan back to Statesboro, and Dan's world suddenly contracted. In California, Dan had been continuously involved in various rehabilitation programs, but programs for people with disabilities were far scarcer in Georgia, and, because of limited funding, they were less easily accessed. Without the kinds of programs he'd engaged in in California, Dan felt his opportunities for improvement slipping away. Shortly after their move, I visited our family in Statesboro while on leave from the Navy, which I had joined in 1979. Half of the household belongings were still in unpacked boxes. Dan escorted me to his new room, where his framed high school diploma already hung on the wall. He pointed to the diploma, then to himself, and spelled, "STUPID." Anguished, I assured him he was not. But clearly Dan needed to be actively participating in programs that helped him work toward specific goals. He longed to recapture his sense of normalcy and increase his ability to move through the world independently, in order to feel that he wasn't completely sidelined.

Still, Dan received a boost he sorely needed when he obtained his Georgia driver's license that summer. And he was thrilled when he applied for and was accepted into a program at the Grier Institute for Rehabilitation. With great relief and soaring expectations, Dan entered the Institute for evaluation and rehabilitation in February of 1983.

Dan's primary goal, upon arriving at Grier, was to engage in vocational rehabilitation—to pinpoint work he could do, and to train in the skills he would need to do it. A job and an income were foundational to his identity as a responsible, productive, independent young adult, an identity that had been severely damaged by his accident. After three apparently constructive weeks in the Institute's Medical Unit, where professionals evaluated his aptitudes and initiated a therapeutic program designed to improve his employment prospects, Dan was transferred to the Vocational Rehabilitation Unit. Four days later, my parents received a call, demanding that they come pick up their son immediately; he had been ejected from the program. Despite my parents' efforts to learn why he was no longer welcome at Grier, they were refused an explanation. The next morning, Mom and Dad made the five-hour car trip to retrieve Dan. They found him alone in his room, desolate, not knowing why he was being forced to leave. Not only was no one available for my parents to ask, but no one was present even to guide them through the check-out process; the unit was deserted, except for Dan. They finally tracked down a custodian and left Dan's room key with him.

Dan had pinned his hopes at qualifying for useful work on the program at Grier. His TBI never has affected the high bar he sets for himself in terms of establishing goals and then putting everything he has into accomplishing them. To have failed despite his best efforts was demoralizing. But to have been summarily terminated from the program—rejected without explanation by an institution that presumably had been established specifically to help people in his situation—was a blow not only to his hopes of reaching a key goal but also to his sense of himself as a valuable and valued member of society. He had acquired severe impairments, yes—and so he required professional assistance to fulfill whatever potential remained to him for reintegrating into that society. He was working as hard as he could to be useful, but he had been told, in effect, that he was unworthy of continued help. In fact, he apparently had been deemed unworthy even of an explanation of what he lacked to finish the program.

What had caused this summary ejection? According to the Institute's records, obtained months later, several days before his eviction Dan moved his truck from one parking lot to another without informing or gaining permission from Grier staff, who for a tense half-hour believed him missing. He didn't know that he needed permission to go outside, however briefly. When the situation was discussed with him, according to the report, he "seemed aware of the responses of staff and his action and indicated that he was amused." Apparently, the staff was affronted by his reaction, but the grounds of his amusement wouldn't have been their alarm per se, but rather that their alarm seemed so overblown to him: so much ado about so little. (I had the same reaction to an analogous situation in boot camp.)

I suspect, as well, that while at Grier Dan had experienced one or more of his anger outbursts. In addition to the Institute's initial description of him as "alert, friendly, and cooperative . . . [with] a good sense of humor," his patient history includes the warning, "he has periodic tantrums when frustrated and may act out aggressively at such times." There is no mention of the connection between his "tantrums"—a word that suggests immaturity as well as willfulness—and his TBI, or to the general prevalence of that issue among survivors of severe TBI. And given that both elevated emotional levels and disruptions to customary routines increase the likelihood of outbursts, Dan's high expectations for improvement coupled with the unfamiliar environment and daily regimen of Grier heightened his susceptibility to episode triggers. In other words, the intensity of his goals and the changes in his surroundings and activities likely ignited the very behavior that resulted in his expulsion from the place he had counted on for help.

Still, Dan's Grier records contained no mention of disturbances to staff other than the truck reparking incident. Whether this transgression or his anger outbursts spurred his abrupt dismissal, our parents were not given any information. They tried for weeks, without success, both to obtain an explanation and to get Dan readmitted into the program. It may seem odd that, following the crushing rejection he had just experienced, he wanted to return to Grier, but there didn't seem to be any other avenue for moving his life forward. This extensive excerpt from a letter Mom wrote as a last-ditch appeal to the executive director of the Institute in March conveys the emotional aftermath (for my parents as well as for Dan) of his experience at Grier:

> [W]e have the feeling that all of the principals in this situation, excepting those in the Medical Unit, wish we would just go away. And if a life were not at stake, perhaps we would.
>
> My husband and I both have to work; therefore, Danny is left every morning to spend the day alone in the house feeling useless and directionless. He has pride, and he is humiliated by his situation, by his mother and father productively engaged while he is stalled, going nowhere. . . . He is anxious to be useful. He still has a good mind—logical, clear, rational. He is responsible and conscientious, and I am *convinced* that there is a place for him in this world where he can contribute—can work and feel useful. It is a matter of his receiving help towards that goal. . . .
>
> I am appealing to you to help us to cut through red tape, bureaucracy, apathy, whatever is barring the door to Danny. We have here a young man who does not want to collect government checks for the rest of his life; he desperately wants to work. And isn't that vocational

rehabilitation's reason for being? Dan will not be as easy to train as a less seriously handicapped person. But someone with skill and patience and caring will find in Danny a willing and cooperative student. Please help.

Although Dan was never readmitted to Grier, Mom's letter did secure an apology and a group conference. The upshot was, however, that Grier wasn't equipped to help people with Dan's disabilities—people with TBI. Mom told me that some years later the facility added rehabilitative treatment options for people with brain injuries. Just not in time to help Dan.

My brother's experience at Grier was the first instance of what would become a recurring motif in his life over the ensuing decades: most people engaged in the American healthcare system don't understand, and are therefore ill-equipped to help, survivors of severe TBI. Over the years, Dan's TBI typically has been (inaccurately) viewed and treated as either deficient intelligence or dementia. There are, of course, entire worlds of difference among these conditions, but the needs, behaviors, and expectations of those occupying these different classes of impairment have been *routinely* misunderstood by care providers at nearly every step. Dan's impairments and competencies differ from those of someone with Down's syndrome or Alzheimer's disease, and the resultant distinctions in capabilities result in problems that require different expectations, approaches, and responses. For example, treating Dan as though he is cognitively incompetent exacerbates his TBI-related explosive episodes, triggering a high percentage of the rage events that over the years have separated him further from strangers, acquaintances, and those charged with his care. This lack of understanding broadens rejection and deepens his social isolation, reducing his opportunities for belongingness. For decades, it has been a vicious cycle: mischaracterization—rage—mischaracterization—rage—mischaracterization. And it is an insufficiently understood, under-appreciated fact that our need for social nourishment is as integral to an acceptable life as is our need for physical sustenance. Furthermore, for people whose physical needs must be tended to by others, their degree of social connection may literally determine how and how long they live, and how they die.

★ ★ ★

Dan's catastrophic fall on the concrete corridor at Troy High School, in which he cracked the plastic plate that had replaced the damaged section of his skull, erased much of the improvement that he had worked so hard to achieve. In the aftermath of that accident, in fact, the severity of his impairments only increased. In effect, he had suffered a second major TBI.

Medical professionals who deal with TBI commonly acknowledge that every brain injury is to some degree unique, as is every survivor. The exact nature of aftereffects is determined by such factors as the location, angle, and force of impact that determine the precise areas of the brain that are affected. Other variables include whether the wound is open, meaning that the injury breaks the skull and penetrates the brain, or closed, when the skull remains intact; the person's age and overall health at the time of the accident; the pre-injury complexity of the individual's already-established neurological pathways and the brain's degree of "plasticity"—its organic ability to reorganize disrupted pathways to create new ones; and the length of time before the person receives medical treatment, and with what degree of expertise. Finally, the singular traits that defined the survivor's premorbid (pre-accident) personality—however much it may have been altered by the injury—serve as a baseline for approaches, resources, and strategies in handling post-injury challenges.

Despite the singularity of each survivor's injury, however, there are neurological impairments, disorders, and syndromes that so commonly arise from TBI that they might be considered "normal" ramifications of brain injury.[2] Some background explanation of the conditions that resulted from Dan's TBI over forty years ago will help contextualize and inform his story. (And at least some of these descriptions will resonate with many other TBI survivors, their families, and their care providers.)

Diffuse Axonal Injury

When someone experiences an injury severe enough to be classified as a TBI, even a mild one, damage occurs not only at points of impact but also throughout the entire brain. As neuropsychiatrist Warren Lux explains, "When the head is accelerated and decelerated abruptly in space, particularly when accompanied by a torsional head movement, strain forces are applied to nerve fibers (axons) throughout the brain."[3] As a result, the brain's axons, which conduct impulses from one cell to another, may be stretched, twisted, or snapped, leaving the survivor with a condition called *diffuse axonal injury* (DAI). In a number of ways, such changes to axons predictably alter the brain's electrochemistry. DAI often occurs in areas completely unaffected by direct force or penetration, and so may impact the entire brain. Consequently, in addition to direct damage done to tissues in specific regions, widespread micro-injuries to axons produce an additional array of deficits and difficulties, including some of those discussed below.

Hemiplegia

The difficulties Dan faces as a result of hemiplegia, or paralysis on one side of the body, don't require much explanation: due to tissue damage in certain areas of the brain that regulate motor control, he can't do anything that requires the use of both hands, both arms, both feet, or both legs. But the sheer number of activities that can only be conducted by using both right and left extremities is extensive. Consider how much we do in a day that requires the use of both hands: washing them, clipping our nails, cutting our food with a knife, using scissors or a can opener, sewing on buttons, pouring milk into a glass with one hand while steadying the glass with the other . . . the list is practically endless. Rising from a chair, crossing a room, turning over in bed—with half of the body immobilized, many quotidian activities become prohibitively difficult, if not impossible.

Besides these physical restrictions of movement, the reactions of others to Dan's paralysis, and even to his wheelchair or to the braces he wears on his arm and wrist, can be at least as debilitating as the hemiplegia itself. Not infrequently, strangers gawk at him as though he's not quite human, while others conspicuously shun him, denying him the baseline social acceptance we routinely offer to the strangers we encounter over the course of a day.

Aphasia and Dysarthria

In 2003, while interviewing Dan as part of my research for postgraduate work in communication studies, I asked him if, given the opportunity to restore one, and only one, of his abilities, which he would choose. Without missing a beat, he spelled, "SPEAK."

I suspected as much, and I understood why. Although each of his impairments is difficult to live with, his inability to speak has had the most global effects on his life. Language proficiency is linked to nearly every aspect of daily living. Aside from the purely instrumental use of language to get things done, we use speech to communicate our desires, interests, ideas, histories, affinities, affiliations, and—perhaps most important of all—our intellectual and social competence, through spoken conversation we share with others. In short, we communicate ourselves—who we believe ourselves to be and how we want others to see us—and engage with others through speech.

Expressive aphasia, the condition that interferes with Dan's ability to produce language, severely restricts his functional use of language. Thankfully, he can still understand everything that is said to him—I can hardly imagine the nightmare of losing that ability, which some aphasics do—but he can generate only single words (basic nouns and adjectives) in isolation; he can't produce the connections between words that create phrases or sentences. He is similarly restricted in his ability to write and, somewhat mysteriously, to read; although he can understand books when they are read to him, on his own he's unable to make sense of the sentences they contain. He can read individual words in abbreviated pieces like lists, signs, labels, and menus, but the sea of sentences in essays and books make no sense to him.

The communicative difficulties caused by Dan's aphasia are compounded by dysarthria, a neurological problem that hampers the movement and coordination of his tongue and lips. So while he can cognitively produce single words, he can't articulate them.

Fortunately, spoken language is not the only tool that people use to communicate. Dan is uncommonly adept with facial expressions and creative gestures. And because he still has command of single words, he's able to use the manual alphabet ("fingerspell") and use a letter board or speaking keyboard. None of these methods work well over the phone, however; fingerspelling and letter boards are strictly visual media, and the speaking keyboard requires proper positioning and renders certain consonants indistinguishable through telephony.[4] His preferred method of communicating through the phone is a system we ourselves devised that we call "alphabetting": I slowly run through each letter of the alphabet, giving him time to emit a sound when I call out the letter he wants to convey. It's a slow process, since each letter of the word he's spelling requires a separate pass through the alphabet, but often the time is shortened by the question, "Is the next letter a vowel?" (eliminating the need to call out consonants in that round) and by successful guesswork based on the first few letters of the word and its conversational context. Sometimes, especially if context hasn't yet been established, even when he successfully spells the words he has in mind, his meaning is still difficult to grasp. As a recent example, he spelled the words "DESK," "BEDROOM," "SLEEP," "NO," "BED," "HANDICAP," "CHAIR." For over half an hour, my interpretations circled around the furniture in his room, but I finally connected my thinking to his and arrived at his meaning: "Would you call the nurse's desk for me? I'm in my room and ready to go to sleep, but they're late getting me ready for bed and I can't do it myself—I'm still in my wheelchair." In retrospect, all of the words represented his thinking, but he lacked the verbs and the glue of prepositions, infinitives, and orderly syntax, so that stringing the words together in a way that reconstructed his thoughts was challenging. Still, while alphabetting often requires forbearance from both Dan and me, it's straightforward, reliable (requires no batteries), and accurate.

In short, Dan engages surprisingly well in conversation, provided his communication partner is willing, persistent, and patient. It helps to comprehend the restricted nature of the linguistic world he operates in, and especially to understand that his difficulty with language doesn't mean that he is cognitively incompetent. The thoughts he intends to convey are logical and contextually relevant. When we have trouble establishing his meaning, I know that the problem is rooted in the processes of production, transmission, and reception, not in the quality or pertinence of the ideas themselves.

Unfortunately, not everyone Dan interacts with understands that. Four years after the accident, a vocational rehabilitation specialist who worked briefly with him noted in a report, "Because he is non-verbal his intellectual ability is likely to be underestimated by others who do not know him well." And because he is unable to speak, he can't correct such misapprehensions.

The underestimation of his mental acuity has been a burden Dan has had to carry continuously for over forty years now. Although post-injury he scored within normal limits on a number of cognitive tests (no small accomplishment for someone with a severe language disorder), people he encounters usually assume from his inability to talk that he's mentally incompetent, which degrades both the tone and content of their interactions with him. Most people he interacts with, even if they've been informed that he is not intellectually disabled, tend to slip into "baby talk." Although being spoken to in this way doesn't prevent Dan from being able to convey his instrumental needs, the relational style itself is a problem. It indicates underlying assumptions that put him at a social disadvantage and complicate his efforts to maintain a positive personal and social identity.

The combination of aphasia and dysarthria, then, compromises every aspect of Dan's life. As aphasia specialists Aura Kagan and Nina Simmons-Mackie put it,

> Conversational interaction is *core* to the ability to participate in virtually every realm of adult life. . . . Without the ability to participate in conversation, every relationship, every life role and almost every life activity is at risk.[5]

They add that the effects of severe communication disorders include "an inevitable loss of self-esteem and a profound sense of social isolation."[6] This problem was identified two years postaccident by the psychiatrist who administered Dan's cognitive tests. He reported,

> Dan tends to be uncomfortable in social situations which of course is related to his inability to carry on a conversation in which he vocalizes the words. People tend to underestimate his intellectual functioning, I am sure, and tend to avoid him which makes him feel more isolated than ever.

Consequently, the few relationships Dan shares with those who perceive and appreciate his intelligence are critically important to him. Those close to him allow him to express his individuality and to feel valued as a social and relational partner—absolutely indispensable elements for a satisfying life.

Dysphagia

In addition to dysarthria, Dan has dysphagia, or difficulty swallowing. As a result of these combined impairments, eating and drinking are more than normally difficult (and messier) for him, he's at increased risk of choking, and he drools almost constantly. While the conscious repositioning of his head can lessen the severity of these problems, it doesn't eliminate any of them. And the downward tilt of his head, which over the years increasingly has become its default position, makes holding it upright nearly impossible to maintain for more than minutes at a time.

The practical physiological problems caused by these conditions are burdensome, but their social impact is even more pronounced. While the language impairments of aphasia and dysarthria lead others to underestimate Dan's competence, his messy eating and his drooling compound the effect. In his report, a vocational rehabilitation specialist Dan worked with noted, "Dan's appearance, especially his drooling, conveys an impression of impairment more severe than exists." And Dan is fully, painfully aware of the misjudgments that arise from these aspects of his self-presentation, as well as the social consequences that attend them.

Anosognosia

Anosognosia is an unwieldy, even ugly, word derived from the Greek *a-* meaning *without*, *-noso-* meaning *malady*, and *-gnosis* meaning *knowledge*: *without knowledge of malady*. Anosognosia is a perplexing neurological condition that causes many TBI survivors to be unaware of, or unable to integrate into their self-understanding, the severity of some of their limitations.[7] It distorts survivors' sense of their own capabilities and the full impact of their impairments. Consequently, those with anosognosia may refuse to adopt strategies and treatments that otherwise might help them improve or compensate for deficits, because they regard assistance in those areas as unnecessary. Additionally, because they may not fully grasp their functional limits, they may overreach those limits, resulting in accidents that can cause further injuries—including (but not only) additional brain injury. This syndrome, then, can exacerbate their impairment, in that they refuse various forms of accommodation that might otherwise offset their compromised functioning, and they may take risks that end up worsening their plight.

It's important for those close to TBI survivors to recognize that people with anosognosia are not *refusing* to acknowledge their deficits; they are *unable* to do so, as a result of neurological damage. Both the survivors themselves and everyone who cares for them can be acutely frustrated by anosognosia's effects; survivors feel that family members, medical professionals, and care providers underestimate their abilities and are insultingly overprotective, while those who love or care for them become exasperated when even their most obviously necessary advice is summarily (and sometimes angrily) rejected. It can be difficult in the moment to remember that people with anosognosia aren't *resisting* reasonable suggestions offered in love or professional wisdom, but that they simply don't *perceive* their limitations as others do.

For example, a brain injury may so compromise my neurological signals that, although I have a number of physiological problems that would make me unsafe behind the wheel of a car—a reduction in response times to stimuli, difficulties in motor function, a restricted field of vision—I believe that the problems that limit me are negligible, or temporary and will surely improve in time, or even that my problems have already adequately resolved. When I'm told that I can no longer drive, my assertion that I'm perfectly capable of driving (or soon will be) will be answered by insistence that I'm being unreasonable (why can't I see how obviously my impairments disqualify me for driving?). What I view as an underestimation of my abilities—one that needlessly obstructs my efforts to live a normal life and deprives me of control over it—will frustrate, insult, and anger me. And the more others withhold from me the opportunity to drive (by hiding the car keys, for instance, or by refusing to take me to the licensing bureau for a driving test), the more frustrated, insulted, and angry I will become.

By its very nature, anosognosia (like many other impairments) is exacerbated by American culture's emphasis on *rugged individualism*. The cultural dictate that *we can do whatever we set our minds to*—and therefore that *we, and we alone, are in control of our lives*—often frames the survivor's refusal to accept limitations as perfectly reasonable—indeed, as the only sanctionable perspective. Combined with the anosognosic's basic belief that *I'm not as impaired as you think I am*, subscription to rugged individualism contributes to a catch-22 situation that encourages survivors to resist adaptation to what may be an irremediable new reality. Further fanning the flames, the countless "heartwarming" examples our culture circulates of heroic triumph when people "overcome" their impairments through sheer persistence, strength of character, and force of will transmits a harmful underlying message: *They succeeded because they didn't give up,* and by extension, *If I try hard enough and don't give up, I will succeed.* This perspective translates quite reasonably to the TBI survivor (and not just those who are anosognosic) as *If I don't succeed, I haven't tried hard enough,* or *I've given up too soon.* The upshot: impairment and acceptance of impairment are tantamount to personal failure.

As a consequence, the anosognosic's efforts at rehabilitation may be sabotaged by an inability to (1) acknowledge some of the kinds of rehabilitation that are needed, (2) formulate goals that are reasonably attainable, (3) abandon cherished aims that are no longer within reach, (4) accept necessary adaptations that will help improve quality of life, and (5) implement precautionary measures that will help to prevent further injury. And relationships with others may tested, at times severely, due to irremediable and mutual vexation.

Intermittent Explosive Disorder

At least as much as anosognosia, and arguably more, another unwieldy neurological problem associated with TBI has profoundly impacted Dan's postaccident life: *intermittent explosive disorder* (IED), which Lux describes as "rage attacks, i.e., brief outbursts of extreme anger, associated with agitated, aggressive, and/or violent behavior" that "have a paroxysmal quality and may occur with little or no provocation."[8] While not related to epilepsy, these dramatic outbursts are seizure-like in nature. Their frequency and ferocity vary according to injury severity and to the degree that aggravating environmental or circumstantial triggers are present. Triggers are often difficult for others to pinpoint, and so the rage attacks may seem entirely unprovoked. These events can be appalling and even fearsome in their intensity, and some people may become violent, posing a risk to the safety of the survivor him- or herself and others. Even absent violence, these uncontrolled outbursts are distressing and likely to impose distance between the affected survivor and others—family, friends, and care providers, as well as strangers—who may view the episodes as evidence of fierce irrationality, unintelligibility, or an inherently violent character. Neuropsychologist Henry Prigatano points out that, for some reason the relationships between survivors and their family members that seem to be most disrupted by IED are those between brain-injured adolescent boys or young adult men and their fathers.[9] Certainly, this dynamic was evident in our family, much to my father's mystification and dismay. And yet the degree to which explosive episodes may compromise survivors' relationships more generally should not be underestimated.

As a result, the familial and social consequences of this disorder can be devastating, as the survivor may be viewed as unduly immature (one nurse described Dan's episodes to me as "the kind of tantrum you'd expect from a two-year-old") and treated with disdain, contempt, or fear and shunned by others. The social isolation and sense of personal rejection and lowered self-image caused by such distancing, especially by family members and personal care providers, can seriously compromise the survivor's well-being, both psychologically and even physically. As Dan's experience attests, compromised social connections with caregivers can lead to neglect or even ill-treatment. IED, then, can trigger a powerful backlash, severely undermining survivors' continual efforts to secure dignity and respect, and at times even threatening their health and safety.

Reduction in Cognitive Processing Speed

Dan is indisputably intelligent and fully aware of everything that is said to or around him. However, especially if he's tired, at times his cognitive functions are slower than usual. He may need questions or comments repeated, and his replies may be momentarily delayed as he thinks through his answers or musters the physiological connections needed to formulate or express them. Correctly or not, I attribute this delay to the extensive rerouting of his neurological pathways following his injury, a feat that strikes me as nothing short of miraculous. However, even though the time lapse between stimulus and response is brief—measurable in mere seconds—it can result in his interactant pressing him for an answer before he is able to give one, with each prod distracting him and causing further delay. Pushed too insistently, he may become frustrated and then angry at what feels to him like undue impatience. In fact, this dynamic can trigger IED episodes and all the negative social consequences that tend to follow in their wake. Without the understanding that Dan occasionally needs extra moments—just a bit more patience—to generate a response, interactions can devolve into situations that are unpleasant for everyone, and that can lead to further social rejection and isolation for him.

Those are the primary neurological impairments that Dan has dealt with on a daily basis for more than forty years. Clearly, the pragmatic functional challenges they pose are serious and at times perilous. And yet their most significant consequences are social. From the moment he regained full consciousness after his accident, Dan has persistently struggled to rebuild a life that is as normal as he can possibly make it. Regrettably, his ability to engage in a number of activities he would enjoy has been curtailed by his impairments. But, more consequentially, the fundamental intangibles that we all yearn for—the essentials we require to feel "normal," like acceptance, friendship, love, and belongingness—have also all too often proven unobtainable for him, beyond his reach no matter how far he stretches.

The elusiveness of positive social relationships is one of the most common consequences of brain injury, and one of the most damaging. Yet Dan, like many other TBI survivors, remains fully capable of both receiving and giving the gifts of acceptance, friendship, love, and belongingness when given a chance. And, as is true for all of us, the more chances he's given, the more normal his life becomes.

★ ★ ★

Following his unceremonious dismissal at the Grier Institute, Dan was at loose ends. Local programs for brain-injured people were nonexistent; rehabilitation programs in general were scarce. He and my parents met with administrators of an organization established in Statesboro for people with developmental disabilities that was in the process of creating a vocational rehabilitation program for its clients. While Dan didn't fit the typical profile of these clients, whose vocational challenges were primarily cognitive rather than physical or communicative, he desperately wanted job training, and its personnel agreed to enter him into their sheltered work program as soon as it was established. In the meantime, they suggested that he participate in their outreach program, with the goal of providing some social contact with someone other than his parents. While he didn't feel that he fit well into the developmentally disabled community, Dan was hungry for a sense of belonging that extended beyond family. He asked to participate in both the outreach program and the vocational training when available. Two staffers promised to be in touch with him, but neither Dan nor our parents ever heard from them again.

Mom repeatedly attempted to contact someone at the organization, but no one was ever available to speak to her when she called, and nobody returned her calls when she left messages. In a letter to the program director, she expressed her exasperation:

> In our association with agencies we are consistently disappointed and let down. I don't think we expect too much; we expect *something*, though. People make promises and don't keep them. . . .
>
> Waiting for someone or something that never happens is depressing, and being neglected or ignored as though it didn't make any difference whether promises are kept, is hard on the ego. . . . Evasion and silence are degrading and insulting. I am reluctantly reaching the conclusion that *no* agency anywhere is going to do anything to help Dan.

This passage reveals the desperation and desolation caused by a lack of belonging—by having been socially judged as someone unworthy of time, attention, or inclusion. Social exclusion impacts not only the person being excluded but also that person's family—parents, siblings, children—as another passage from Mom's letter demonstrates:

> I am bitter and full of despair because agencies whose sole purpose for being is to help the handicapped are, without fail, failing us. I do not know what to do next nor where to turn. If you by any chance have any suggestions or information, I would appreciate your response.

The response to Mom's letter was a referral to a neurosurgeon. Within a year, Mom would be writing various letters to lawyers—as well as one to the CBS TV show *Sixty Minutes*—in an unsuccessful attempt to expose that neurosurgeon as an unscrupulous opportunist, hoping to prevent the potential victimization of other people with TBI and their families. But as of the spring of 1984, our family had not yet experienced the kind of trauma inflicted by a scoundrel who would take advantage of a young man's desperation for normalcy—a normalcy critical not only because of its functional advantages but also because of its correlation with identity, inclusion, and belonging.

Notes

1. Roy F. Baumeister and Mark R. Leary, "The Need to Belong: Desire for Interpersonal Attachments as a Fundamental Human Motivation," *Psychological Bulletin* 117, no. 3 (1995): 497–529. doi: 10.1037/0033-2909.117.3.497; Geoff WillDonald and Mark R. Leary, "Why Does Social Exclusion Hurt? The Relationship between Social and Physical Pain," *Psychological Bulletin* 131, no. 2 (2005): 202–23. doi: 10.1037/0033-2909.131.2.202; John T. Cacioppo and William Patrick, *Loneliness: Human Nature and the Need for Social Connection* (New York: W.W. Norton & Company, 2008); Kipling D. Williams, Joseph P. Forgas, and William von

Hippel, *The Social Outcast: Ostracism, Social Exclusion, Rejection, and Bullying* (New York: Psychology Press, 2014); and Kelly-Ann Allen, *The Psychology of Belonging* (London: Routledge, Taylor & Francis Group, 2021).
2. Warren E. Lux, "A Neuropsychiatric Perspective on Traumatic Brain Injury" *The Journal of Rehabilitation Research & Development* 44, no. 7 (2007): 951–62. doi: 10.1682/jrrd.2007.01.0009
3. Lux, 952.
4. For some reason I've not been able to ascertain, Dan dislikes using keyboards that speak entire words or Augmentative and Alternate Communication (AAC) computer devices; he has tried several kinds, rejected them, and isn't interested in trying any others.
5. Aura Kagan and Nina Simmons-Mackie, "Changing the Aphasia Narrative" *The ASHA Leader* 18, no. 11 (2013): 7. doi: 10.1044/leader.fmp.18112013.6
6. Kagan and Simmons-Mackie, 8.
7. Lux, "A Neuropsychiatric Perspective," 956.
8. Lux, 956.
9. Henry P. Prigatano, *Principles of Neuropsychological Rehabilitation* (New York: Oxford University Press, 1999), 81.

4 Dan's Life
1984–2006

On June 19, 1984, Dan and Mom arrived at St. Benedict Hospital in the Bronx, in New York City. Mom handed nearly $13,000 (equivalent to about $36,000 in 2022) in certified checks, as instructed, to the office of neurosurgeon James Strauss. Dan had an appointment with Dr. Strauss later that afternoon for a consultation to determine if he was a good candidate for an experimental procedure that might restore, or at least improve, some of the neurological integrity he had lost. The procedure consisted of the implantation of an electronic transmitter in Dan's back, which would then be manipulated by an external transmitter with variable frequency and pulse width settings. Electrical impulses would be sent along his spinal cord to stimulate nerves, with the expectation of improving their ability to function.

Dr. Strauss determined that Dan was a prime candidate for the surgery, and he implanted the transmitter the next morning. In a nine-page document, Mom recorded the sequence of events leading up to and following the surgery. In sum, Dr. Strauss failed to provide until *after* the surgery documentation that said, "Spinal cord stimulation has not been shown to be of value in the treatment of dysfunctions due to brain lesions or tumors." Mom writes,

> This statement was like a blow between the eyes. I felt that we had been "had," and that everyone but us knew this from the start. It was one thing to be part of an experimental procedure that had a reasonable chance of success. It was quite another to subject Dan to this surgery, to raise his hopes that his life was going to be improved, to relieve us of roughly $13,000, when there was no chance that this procedure would work with Dan. I had not been looking for any such evidence, but here it was. . . . Had this information been made available to us prior to the surgery, we would not have followed through with it. . . .

I went to [Dan's primary care doctor] and asked him if Dan had "brain lesions." I knew the answer, but I wanted confirmation. He said, "Of course Dan has brain lesions. Anyone who was kicked in the head as he was has a large area of brain lesions."

Mom's subsequent efforts to contact Dr. Strauss were ignored, despite his pre-surgery assurance that, because the procedure was experimental and detailing the outcome was valuable research information, Dan would be part of a two-year follow-up study. The last time Dan saw Dr. Strauss was in a hallway the day after his operation, when the doctor hurriedly wrote Dan a prescription for an antibiotic and left discharge orders at the desk for the following morning—four days earlier than planned. Neither Dan nor Mom ever saw or heard from Dr. Strauss again.

Not incidentally, the antibiotic Dr. Strauss prescribed proved to be related to penicillin, despite Mom's emphatic warning during the consultation that Dan was severely allergic to penicillin, that he had nearly died of anaphylactic shock in childhood and was warned that he never should take the drug again. By early evening, Dan's eyes had begun to swell, and he was having difficulty breathing. Mom's record of that night at the hospital reads, "Dan continued to get worse. He began to cry he was so frightened. . . . [H]e kept spelling 'blind' on his fingers." A nurse called Dr. Strauss at 6:30 p.m., relaying Dan's condition and Mom's urgent request that he come, but no doctor saw Dan in the hospital that night. The nurse told Mom that Dan was obviously having an extreme reaction to the drug, and she promised not to administer any more of it.

In a letter to a lawyer a year later, Mom wrote,

> I believe that James M. Strauss has used my son and me for his personal gain. I believe he has made no effort to follow up because he already knew before he did the surgery what the outcome would be. He has taken advantage of my handicapped son, and Dr. Strauss's opportunism in such a situation is particularly unconscionable. He has also relieved my husband and me of all of our savings. In addition, my son is walking around with useless material implanted in his body. . . .
>
> I assure you that we would have had no complaint had the surgery been done in good faith and had simply failed. For nearly seven years we have been involved with doctors and hospitals. Over that length of time, accidents due to negligence, etc. have occurred. Sometimes surgeries, procedures, therapies which we had hoped would work have not. But in all cases, the doctors and medical personnel have been honorable people with good intentions. This experience with

Dr. Strauss is the first time that I have felt "used," have felt that we encountered a patently dishonest doctor.

I have no reason to doubt Mom's conclusion that Dr. Strauss exploited my brother and our parents; in fact, her careful documentation supports it. Such exploitation is only committable by someone who feels no connection to those they target. Dan's pain and harsh disappointment, like Mom and Dad's disillusionment and depleted savings account, were by-products of Dan and our parents being viewed, not as people who matter, but as easy fruit, ripe for the picking.

Exactly one year after Dr. Strauss implanted the transmitter in Dan's back, Mom and Dad were approved for a loan that paid for Dan to have another surgery, this time at Emory University Hospital, where surgeons removed the useless equipment that had turned a handy profit for Dr. Strauss.

★ ★ ★

Just before his twenty-sixth birthday in March 1986, Dan went to the Department of Motor Vehicles in Statesboro for a routine renewal of his driver's license, which was scheduled for expiration. His driving record was good; he'd received his first ticket in Georgia the year before when he bumped into a car ahead of him at a red light. The bump was so slight that no damage was done and so no insurance claim was filed, and the judge waived the traffic fine.

However, Mom, Dad, Dave, and I had recently been complaining to Dan about his driving, which was becoming erratic. Whenever the issue was raised, Dan angrily insisted that he drove perfectly well, consummately illustrating a TBI-related disorder that we had never heard of and had no term for but which I would later learn: anosognosia. His defense of his driving seemed mysterious to us, an instance of willful and illogical denial; we knew he was scrupulously honest, and we didn't understand at the time that Dan was neurologically incapable of putting together what was, for us, clear evidence of a decline in his driving ability. Instead, he dismissed a series of near-misses—caroms into curbs, swerves toward ditches, various close calls—as inconsequential, claiming that since they hadn't resulted in accidents, they didn't indicate a noteworthy problem. In his view, we were being alarmist and judgmental, underestimating his competence. We occasionally argued with him about it, but we didn't do more than that—not simply because our insistence on this point typically triggered rage episodes but because driving was of monumental importance to Dan. We all felt that he'd lost more than enough already, and we were reluctant—despite potentially disastrous consequences—to impose more loss. Dan always drove slowly, and as carefully as he could. We were struggling to find a safe resolution to this problem that wouldn't add yet another crushing loss to Dan's long list of losses.

When Dan went to the DMV for a perfunctory license renewal that spring, the clerk took one look at him and required him to take a road test. The examiner was dissatisfied with the results and filed his license for review by the Medical Advisory Board. I have no record of how Dan's performance failed to meet her standards, but he couldn't have done too badly; she did approve a temporary permit, and in May he received his regular license in the mail. He was elated, believing that the threat to his driving privileges was over.

However, in June, Dan received a letter from the Medical Advisory Board, requiring certification of his competency from two different doctors and a recent electroencephalogram (EEG) report, all of which were submitted in July. The evaluations of both doctors were positive, indicating their conviction that he was capable of driving responsibly.

In August, Dan took another road test with the same examiner who had sent his license to the Board for review in March. During the test, she refused to allow him to use the adaptive steering knob which made his driving considerably easier and safer and was required for him to drive in California. The evaluator deemed his reflexes were too slow, dismissing his driving record with the remark that he must have been lucky for the past four years. She arranged for him to take another road test that same afternoon with the chief examiner in Swainsboro, thirty-five miles away.

In September, the Medical Advisory Board revoked his license.

In October, Dad wrote a letter of appeal on Dan's behalf, using the first person to express his son's perspective:

> I drove the thirty-five miles to Swainsboro. By then I was tired and nervous and demoralized. I decided that, since Ms. Jones [the examiner in Statesboro] had criticized my "slow reflexes," I would try to execute my turns quickly and impress the examiner. During the test I therefore tried to make a turn much faster than I usually do and I sideswiped a parked car. Damage to the car and to my truck was minimal (scratched paint), but this error constituted failure, of course, and I surrendered my license at the examiner's request.

Although Dad felt that Dan's driving was becoming at times unsafe and urged Dan to voluntarily stop driving, he fought for the reinstatement of his son's license. Some might consider that decision hypocritical, or irresponsible, or even irrational, but to Dad it was simply a matter of fairness.

If Dan had been able to write or speak, he would have fought for himself. He had a right to explain his viewpoint and defend his stance, but he lacked the means. So Dad became his means. In his packet appealing the Board's decision, Dad explained the practical importance of driving to Dan, the reason that no one in the family had proactively sought to take him off the road: "By revoking his driver's license, the Department of Public Safety has drastically undercut Dan's efforts to live as normally and independently as possible and in effect has sentenced him to house arrest for life."

As a result of Dad's efforts, a hearing was scheduled, but the revocation was upheld. Still, Dan was not dissuaded. Some months later, in the summer of 1987, he completed a driving course at a Savannah high school, presented his certificate to the DMV, and requested another road test. His efforts and persistence were rewarded: he regained his license. However, the reprieve proved temporary. One rainy night, he lost control of his truck on a deserted highway and slid into a ditch. The highway patrolman who responded to the accident confiscated his license. Considering the struggle it had been to regain his license this last time, Dan recognized the odds against another successful battle.

Dan was absolutely devastated by the loss of his driver's license—as we had known he would be. For the first time in his life, despite the various catastrophes and monumental disappointments visited upon him in the nine years since the accident in Chelsea, Dan was so distraught that our parents were afraid to leave him alone, afraid of what he might do. For nearly a month, the family's minister and his wife sat with Dan for the hours that Mom taught her college classes until the semester ended. Mom said that Dan lay in bed for hours, hardly moving, and when she would check on him, he would fingerspell, "DIE."

★ ★ ★

After losing his driver's license the first time in March of 1986, the range of Dan's life shrank. Barely able to walk and living in a town without public transportation, Dan passed his days by himself in the studio apartment appended to Mom and Dad's house. No longer could he spend his afternoons downtown or at the mall, grocery shopping or getting a haircut or buying the occasional birthday gift, nor could he drive himself to medical or dental appointments, or to weekly maintenance therapy sessions at the local hospital. He was unable to get himself to Ron Lewis's horse ranch only five miles away, where he had been receiving rehabilitative riding instruction that helped him maintain his muscle tone and balance—and put him in the company of horses, which he had missed. The loss of his driving privileges narrowed the scope of his life to long days in front of the TV, waiting for Mom and Dad to come home from work.

Our parents continued to scout for programs that would offer Dan opportunities to enrich his life. We were all thrilled when, that November, Dan was awarded a six-month scholarship to The Palms Rehabilitation Center, a facility in Florida with therapeutic programs that focused on residential community re-entry for brain-injured adults. Dan approached his stay at The Palms with a renewed sense of hope and direction. He was eager to work at recovering abilities and skills that would allow him to live more fully and, of primary importance, independently. Not least of all, he hoped to be able to drive again. The overall outlook seemed encouraging. In a letter to The Palms on December 29, one month to the day after Dan had entered the center, Dad wrote, "We were impressed by the interest shown by each staff member and with the general objectives for improving Dan's future."

While the therapists treated Dan well and did their best to help him, in the end, his work at The Palms accomplished little. In their initial assessment, Dan's rehabilitation team wrote, "The two functional outcome goals are: 1) Supervised independent living; and 2) vocational/avocational exploration and possible training in his community of Statesboro, Georgia." In their discharge report six months later, the same team wrote,

> Return to live with family in a supervised living environment. . . . It is recommended that Danny receive services in a highly structured, well organized day activities program due to his physical limitations and possible injury to himself if unsupervised.

After half a year of full-time rehabilitation, and despite his unflagging efforts, Dan's goals of living on his own and finding work he could do had been pronounced unrealistic—even potentially dangerous—by The Palms's rehabilitation team. Dan's return to Statesboro in April, no closer to independence than he had been in November, was another disappointment, another defeat, that he surely experienced as one more judgment, one more dismissal.

★ ★ ★

The months between the loss of Dan's license and his acceptance to The Palms had been difficult, but Mom described the period that followed his discharge from The Palms in April of 1987 as "hellish." The inescapable fact was that Dan, who had left home at eighteen to work his way through the world, was now a man in his late twenties, unemployed—and, what was worse, officially declared unemployable—and still living with his parents, in a studio apartment appended to *their* house. And the disappointment of The Palms followed closely on the heels of the permanent loss of his license. Dan's sense of himself as a functioning member of society, as someone who could contribute, someone who *belonged*, was painfully countered by forced dependence and a string of losses and perceived failures. His misery was deepened by the prospect that what remained of his lifetime would be a succession of interminable empty days, devoid of meaning or purpose or the kinds of relationships and connections that most of us take for granted.

In the bleak period following Dan's release from The Palms, his customary patience and tolerant good nature all but vanished. The accretion of frustrations and disappointments exacerbated both the frequency and the severity of his IED outbursts, which often culminated in shattered glass and splintered furniture as he lashed out in fury against his despair. These episodes were usually directed toward Mom and Dad, who could no more escape their situation than Dan could escape his. All three were trapped, with nowhere else to go, and without any solution they could think of that might alleviate their intolerable circumstances.

One of Dan's major problems was that, despite his continuous efforts at rehabilitation aimed at improving and restoring lost abilities and skills, his physical condition was slowly but inexorably deteriorating. Some therapists posited that, in trying to do everything he possibly could for himself, Dan simply pushed his body too hard, and it was wearing out. Also, his occasional falls, while not appearing to be serious events when considered singly, may have been incrementally compromising his ability to function. Whatever the cause, or causes, Dan was experiencing progressively more difficulty.

In the years that followed Dan's initial accident, family members would frequently "buddy-walk" with him: Dan would put his arm around his walking partner's neck, leaning for support, and they would move together toward his desired destination. As his physical capabilities waned, however, Dan's buddies were performing increasingly more of the work. This duty mainly fell to Dad, since Mom was no longer able to support much of Dan's weight, and both Dave and I lived out of state. As Dad got older, the physical strain on him intensified, eventually resulting in a hernia. Still, as soon as he recuperated from the resultant surgery, he resumed buddy-walking duties.

For years, physical therapists and rehabilitation specialists, as well as family members, had pressed Dan to use a wheelchair. And for years, he flatly refused—indeed, he was infuriated by the suggestion. For Dan, a wheelchair represented capitulation, a step further away from normalcy, which he was still continually striving to reach. But the situation worsened; in 1988, at sixty-two years old, Dad was diagnosed with cancer. His surgery was extensive and permanently debilitating: Dad's buddy-walking days were over. Although Dan continued for a while to use a walker, moving across a room was slow and laborious, and he was falling with growing frequency.

The issue was resolved at last, with great discomfiture, on Dave's wedding day in 1989. Following the ceremony, Dave and his new wife held a reception in a large hall adjoining the church sanctuary. In the excitement, as friends and family escorted the couple toward their reception, Dan was forgotten, abandoned in a pew near the altar. Though his absence was noted within a few minutes and he was soon brought into the reception hall, the time he passed alone in the sanctuary, his family celebrating without him, made him feel utterly brushed aside, unvalued.

At Dave's house that evening, Dan was still upset. Dave apologized but also pointed out with some exasperation that we—and especially he himself—had been understandably distracted, and that had Dan been using a wheelchair rather than relying on Dave for buddy-walking, he could have joined in the celebration at will, instead of depending on others (specifically, Dave) to transport him from place to place. Though Dan was initially furious, the lesson hit home: a wheelchair would boost, rather than hinder, his participation in life activities. Rather than signaling resignation, a wheelchair would help him move through the world more independently.

The battle was over. Dan was soon zipping from place to place in a new motorized wheelchair, giving the lie to the common view that people are "confined" to wheelchairs. In fact, wheelchairs liberate.

Dan's wheelchair empowered him with some of the freedom and independence he had craved for years. In April of 1991, he signed a one-year lease with Oliver Place, a government-subsidized apartment building for Social Security recipients located in Savannah, fifty-five miles from Statesboro. Dan planned to establish his independence by living alone for a year, just to prove he could do it; when the year was over, he expected to return to his apartment in Mom and Dad's house. Our parents viewed Dan's upcoming period in Savannah with some trepidation, but mostly with relief. They urgently needed a respite from the relentless emotional conflagrations that had been consuming all three of their lives in recent years.

As it turned out, Dan lived at Oliver Place for eleven years and four months. His life in Savannah was solitary, but he gained the greater independence and sense of self-reliant adulthood that he so desired, which he was unwilling to relinquish when the year was over. Although his efforts at sociability were still severely curtailed by his communication difficulties, and he characterizes his life in Savannah as "LONELY," he was less isolated than he had been in Statesboro. He attended St. Paul's Episcopal Church every Sunday and met with a disability support group at St. James Catholic Church each month. While most of his fellow residents at Oliver Place were elderly, he shared a pleasant acquaintanceship with many of them—they were friendly, familiar faces—and several of the men joked with him when they met in the lobby or passed by in the hall. Additionally, he had a succession of paid buddy-walkers, as well as contact with Oliver Place staff members, dentists, doctors, grocery and retail store clerks, and others—the sorts of informal interactions that help us move smoothly and sociably through our lives. Some of these encounters were marred by negative reactions from others, but many people were friendly, especially those for whom Dan became a familiar face.

Once Dave returned to Georgia, moving to an Atlanta suburb that was a four-hour drive from Savannah, he spent time with Dan as often as he could, and even occasionally took him to momentous events like the Kentucky Derby in Lexington and the Preakness Stakes at Pimlico Downs. Less frequently, I visited from my home in North Carolina. Mom and Dad made weekly trips from Statesboro to visit, treating Dan to restaurant meals and helping him grocery shop, until shortly before Dad's death in November of 2000. Afterward, Mom continued to make the weekly trek to visit, but, now in her seventies and dealing with emphysema, she was unable to take Dan out to eat or help him at the grocery store. Several members of a men's group at his church—one faithful friend in particular—assumed some of those tasks, and with the help of Georgia Friends, a social services agency that provided assistants for buddy-walking, transportation to and from health care appointments, and occasional grocery shopping expeditions when no one else was available, Dan got along fairly comfortably. After all, he was enmeshed in a community, a set of relationships that extended his sense of belonging. Not surprisingly, he still views his time at Oliver Place as one of the most rewarding periods of his adult life.

★ ★ ★

Dan's residence at Oliver Place came to an abrupt, unceremonious end in July 2002, when one sunny Saturday afternoon, he fell down in his kitchen. Though he tried for hours, he was unable to reach his wheelchair or to pull himself up. The emergency call button on the wall was maddeningly close, but he couldn't reach it. No one heard his cries for help.

The assistant who was scheduled to buddy-walk with him on Sunday never showed up. When Oliver Place staff found Dan late Monday morning, he was rushed by ambulance to the emergency room unconscious, severely dehydrated, in renal failure, and nearly dead.

Dan was traumatized both physically and emotionally. Lying on the floor in his kitchen, he believed he would die, and he almost did. His independence had betrayed him, proving to some degree illusory. Mom, Dave, and I were horrified. Since his accident, Dan had ceaselessly battled to achieve as much autonomy as he was able to wrest from his largely uncooperative body; our job, as we saw it, was to discover and protect the fine line between supporting his efforts for independence and preventing him from overextending himself and causing further injury—a job complicated by his anosognosia. From the very beginning, he was infuriated by our efforts to do anything for him that he felt he could do for himself, and over the years we became accustomed to—though never comfortable with—standing by for long, breathless minutes as Dan, with painstaking slowness and utmost concentration, accomplished some physical feat that he simply didn't seem capable of. We constantly wrangled with our own unease over the risks Dan would take, trying to cope with our own fears in an attempt to champion Dan's pursuit of his ever-diminishing dreams, to refrain from breaking his spirit or simply enraging him through overprotection. For several years, we all had been noticing his gradual decline, but none of us realized that he was experiencing the level of incapacity that his fall at Oliver Place revealed, in part because, for over a decade, he had proudly managed (though, as it turned out, less smoothly than we had believed) with minimal assistance. And not only had we adapted to the fact that his life involved a high degree of physical struggle, but Dan, unwilling to jeopardize his hard-won independence, hadn't complained about the increased level of hardship he had been facing.

Just two weeks before the nearly fatal fall in his kitchen, Dan had been released from hospital observation following a less serious fall; when he returned to Oliver Place, we assumed his life would resume with the same degree of difficulty—no more, no less—that living his life inherently entailed. However, during this latest hospitalization, his physician discovered bone scarring that suggested a history of untreated fractures. She initially suspected that someone had been physically abusing him, until he managed to convince her that her suspicions were unfounded. We were at least as shocked as the doctor by the fact that Dan had sustained multiple fractures without telling anyone, either because he hadn't realized the extent of his injuries or (more likely) out of fear that he would lose the independence he had been experiencing at Oliver Place.

This latest fall demonstrated to everyone that Dan's life at Oliver Place was unsustainable. Not only was his doctor refusing to release him to return to Oliver Place, but Oliver Place was unwilling to accept him back anyway, since it was now clear that he could no longer safely manage independent living. Dad had died the year before, and because of her own physical challenges, Mom was ill-equipped to care for him at home. Suddenly, Dan had nowhere to go.

Dave spent two hectic weeks driving back and forth from Atlanta to Savannah, meeting with social workers, doctors, and therapists, trying to determine Dan's needs and how best to meet them. Several years earlier, Mom, Dad, Dave, and Dan had scouted various living arrangements in the Atlanta area that would be within driving distance for Dave to visit regularly. Dan was placed on several waiting lists. Each time an opening became available, he was notified and, in each instance, he declined to move, preferring instead to remain at Oliver Place. Dave now contacted each facility, but none had a place for him, and Dan no longer qualified for most of them anyway, since the level of assistance he needed had increased.

Dan's deadline for leaving the hospital was fast approaching. Almost miraculously, a bed at Taylor Heights Health and Rehabilitation Center suddenly became available. The professionals Dave had been meeting with praised Taylor Heights, citing its unusually good record for patient health and longevity. When Dave dropped in unannounced to inspect the facility, staff welcomed him, showing him every area without hesitation. He came away from the visit impressed by the friendliness and professionalism of personnel, pleased with the level of cleanliness and order, and vastly relieved that they were willing to accept Dan immediately, even before receiving the paperwork that confirmed his Medicaid eligibility.

Dan had a place to go at last. And while we were elated that he would be safe and cared for in what was apparently one of the best of all possible nursing homes, there was no avoiding the unhappy fact that Taylor Heights was, in fact, a *nursing home*, whose ranks were almost entirely filled by elderly folks, many of whom were struggling with various stages of dementia. Even those residents who were competent were of our parents', not Dan's, generation. His opportunities for social connection and belonging, diminished because of his various impairments but enlarged by his ties in Savannah, suddenly dwindled. He was deeply disheartened, and no wonder. At the age of forty-two, he was facing the prospect of spending the rest of his life in a nursing home.

★ ★ ★

Dan entered Taylor Heights Health and Rehabilitation Center as a resident in September of 2002. In January, I drove down from my new home in Indiana, where I had moved to marry Dyke the previous summer, to spend a week with Dan at Taylor Heights. My visit was not only familial, although certainly it was that too. I was completing my master's degree with an ethnographic study that put Dan at the heart of my project. My research question was this: given the endless stream of assaults on Dan's sense of himself as a "normal" person—the torrent of seriously compromising physical, emotional, and social experiences that had been part of his daily life for the previous twenty-four years—how had he managed to maintain his identification with his pre-accident normalcy? This question arose because, without a scintilla of doubt, from the moment he regained consciousness, Dan has continued to view himself as fundamentally normal, despite the enormous physical, behavioral, and social challenges he continually confronts. Given prevailing theories at the time of how identity forms and operates, it was a fascinating (and for me, a personally engaging) question, and I gathered plenty of information that enabled me to write a thesis I'm still proud of nearly twenty years later.

Also, however, that visit—my brief but intense immersion into his daily life—had an unintended consequence. It fostered in me a deeper, more radical understanding of and empathy for Dan's point of view. Contrary to our family's hopes for him, Dan emphatically didn't *want* to adapt to life in a nursing home. He felt relegated to what seemed like an extended version of death, walled off from the world of bustling, variegated normalcy, bereft of relationships and activities that genuinely engaged him. Repeatedly over my week-long visit, Dan pleaded with me to get him out of Taylor Heights. By the week's end, I had moved from encouraging him to psychically adjust, to trying to help him move out of Taylor Heights into a community setting.

Despite my heightened understanding of Dan's plight and my desire to help him out of it, making that decision was difficult for several reasons. His impairments, both physical and behavioral, raised the question of how well he would handle increased autonomy and the new social as well as logistical conditions he would confront out in the community. I hoped that he could meet these challenges successfully, but, especially after the revelations about the serious difficulties he'd endured at Oliver Place, I also had doubts. Additionally, Dave had worked hard to find a safe harbor for Dan; I sincerely appreciated his efforts and didn't want to dishonor them or undermine him. But from Dan's perspective, this new level of safety was far too costly, requiring that he surrender his sense of himself as a relatively young man (by nursing home standards) living in the "normal" world, and the forfeiture of any interests he still had or any dreams that he might yet formulate for his future. So while I worried that leaving the safety of Taylor Heights might not work out well for Dan, I worried more about what might happen to him if he stayed. Just as Dad had respected Dan's right to fight for his driver's license and so had written letters on Dan's behalf despite his own reservations, I was moved by what felt to me like Dan's right to pursue a different, potentially more satisfying living arrangement. So at Dan's request, and after several difficult discussions with Dave, I orchestrated, by phone from Indiana over a period of months, Dan's transfer from Taylor Heights into the private home of a care provider who contracted with Georgia Friends. And I held my breath.

★ ★ ★

Dan moved out of Taylor Heights on August 15, 2003. He joined his new care provider Carl, Carl's prepubescent son, and two other new "clients" in Carl's split-level home on a tree-lined street in the Atlanta area. The neighborhood had a peaceful suburban feel, even though it was separated from the heavy urban traffic of I-285 only by a slim stand of trees and hedges. The lower level of the home contained two bedrooms (one of them Dan's), a bathroom, and a spacious living room lined by a wall of sliding glass doors that opened into a large, fenced-in back yard fringed with trees, shrubs, and flowers. It felt like a true home, without the institutional erasure from the rest of the world that was largely what Dan had hoped to escape. At Carl's, Dan had the opportunity to become part of a small but tightly knit social family. By October, he had been measured for a new wheelchair, visited the dentist for the first time in three years, and participated in a number of fun activities, such as bowling, spending a day at Six Flags Over Georgia, and—by far his favorite of the outings—whizzing around in a go-cart. Carl reported that Dan was doing well, learning to be increasingly cooperative and flexible. However, hinting at Dan's ongoing struggle with IED, Carl added, "He still has his moments." He noted one occasion when Dan, after a frustrating training session on a new communication device, had his arm cocked to hurl the $8000 computer at a wall. Fortunately, Carl was able to intervene in time, averting an expensive disaster. (Dan never did accept use of the device; I assume it was returned.) IED was little recognized—and even less well understood—as a predictable syndrome arising from TBI even among caregiving professionals, and neither Carl nor any of our family had ever heard of it; we had only experienced it. Dan's episodic rages in his new home had increasingly deleterious effects, interfering with Carl's genuine desire to provide an extended family for Dan. Because of his anosognosia, Dan underestimated the seriousness of his explosive storms and the impact they had on others—and, consequently, of the damage they did to his relationships and his living circumstances. He didn't realize that living at Carl's was directly dependent on the quality of their relationship and the degree of belonging that arose, or failed to arise, from it.

Adding to the changes Dan experienced in adjusting to his new environment, just before Dan left Taylor Heights, Dave left for Iraq, working for a company that contracted with the Department of Defense to train Iraqi paramilitary forces in combat medicine. As a result, his weekly visits with Dan had been suspended for a year. Dave sent letters, I called at least weekly to check in, and Dyke and I drove down from Indiana every few months, bringing Mom up from Statesboro the few times she was physically able to make the trip. Despite our efforts, Dan lacked the level of family presence he had been accustomed to in previous years. So we were especially grateful to Carl for providing Dan with social as well as physical support. He seemed to genuinely like Dan, and although he continued to note Dan's volatile outbursts, his reports were predominantly positive, emphasizing Dan's increasing integration within his new home. During one of my frequent phone conversations with Carl, I was gratified when he referred to Dan as an important member of "the family I'm putting together," adding, "and it *is* a family." Dan, it seemed, would be receiving the emotional as well as physical support he needed in order to live a more satisfying life.

When Mom died in March 2005, Dan rode with Dave to Statesboro for her memorial service. Even though Mom's health had been declining for months, her death was crushing. All three of us were profoundly grief-stricken, and Carl was saddened by our loss and warmly sympathetic. At this point, we felt as though Carl was an extended part of our own family.

I was therefore dumbfounded when seven weeks later—nineteen months after Dan had moved in with Carl—Georgia Friends called me with the news that Carl had terminated his living arrangement with Dan. The day before, I was told, following one of their customary outings, instead of returning home, Carl surprised Dan by dropping him off, with an overnight bag he had secreted in his trunk beforehand, at another Georgia Friends-contracted home. Dan had received no advance warning that he was being evicted from his home with Carl. He had never before met or even heard mention of the couple in whose house he now found himself. Unable to speak or walk, and with his own family unaware of his whereabouts until Georgia Friends called me the next day, Dan was suddenly and completely adrift.

Carl never communicated with Dan, Dave, or me again. I phoned several times over the next few days but got no answer, and my voicemails were never returned. We were left to guess at the reason for Dan's expulsion from the "family" Carl had put together, whose bonds had proven less durable than we had hoped. I suspected that Carl was no longer willing to deal with Dan's IED rages. He had noted a decrease in their frequency as Dan adjusted to his new situation, but Dan's volatility may have escalated in the aftermath of Mom's death. Losing her was intensely painful for me, and it may well have been even worse for Dan. Although Carl hadn't mentioned any increased behavioral difficulties, I speculated that grief may have intensified Dan's IED.

More than a decade later, I received an official explanation for Dan's expulsion when I came into possession of a five-inch binder containing Carl's records of Dan's various appointments with doctors, dentists, and therapists. The paperwork does contain a few references to Dan's "explosive" temper. But the final straw for Carl seems to have been a different issue. Because of his dysphagia, a speech therapist had ordered that Dan's food be ground, puréed, or cut into very small pieces to lessen his risk of choking. Despite her advisory, Dan was adamant about eating *normal* food, *normally* prepared, just like everyone else's—an expression of anosognosia, as he believed that his dysphagia posed no serious threat and that his ability to live *normally* was being underestimated yet again. The Georgia Friends paperwork includes a statement that Carl had twice performed the Heimlich maneuver on Dan, and he was unwilling to take the chance that Dan might choke to death under his care. I don't know whether or not he ever shared with Dan that compliance with the therapist's recommendations was a condition of remaining in Carl's household, but the morning after his eviction when I spoke with Dan on the phone, his pained bewilderment at the sudden change in his circumstances was as clear as his anxiety and despair.

Certainly, Carl had been in a difficult position. In light of Dan's resistance to the speech therapist's orders, I don't blame Carl for deciding that he was no longer willing to be responsible for Dan's well-being. He had every right to terminate his role as care provider. What I do have difficulty understanding is the cruelty of the *way* he did it—in an instant permanently barring Dan from the place he had considered home for almost two years, and casting him into the hands of total strangers. Dan had no time to prepare, either logistically or emotionally, for his eviction. Neither Dave nor I knew of Carl's plan until after it had been executed, so we were unable to help make alternative arrangements or to provide Dan with any sense of reassurance, stability, protection, or oversight—to help him go *through* it. It may be that Georgia Friends directed Carl to withhold his intentions from Dan (and us) in order to avoid triggering an outburst. But, as unpleasant as Dan's emotional paroxysms could be, the consequences of the worst of them pale in comparison to the distress and anxiety that Carl's actions inflicted on Dan. The abruptness with which he was dumped on the doorstep of strangers drove home at least two lessons: Dan lacked even a modicum of control over his life, and the inclusion he had believed he'd found at Carl's was illusory. In short, Dan felt thoroughly rejected and abandoned when it may have hurt him most, in the aftermath of his mother's death. And after years of seeking relative independence, there was no arguing the fact that he was basically helpless, that there was always the potential that he might have no input over even the most fundamental aspects of his own circumstances. Had Carl intentionally devised a scenario that would make Dan feel rejected, isolated, and utterly disempowered—radically *disabled*—he couldn't have more fully accomplished those ends.

An even marginally functional bond of belonging would have demanded a different solution. The ends may have been the same, but the means Carl used would have been unimaginable.

★ ★ ★

Although his stay in Audra and Marshall's home was originally intended to be only a stopgap, Dan spent a full year there, from April 2005 to April 2006. Dave had returned from Iraq the previous October, so his weekly visits and outings with Dan had resumed, and Dyke and I visited from Indiana every few months. Still, the year is mostly a blank for Dan. Perhaps he remembers little from that period because there was so little to remember.

On Dyke's and my first visit, we toured Dan's quarters—a nicely finished, freshly painted, well-appointed basement with a bedroom, bathroom, and TV sitting room. For the most part, Dan was comfortable. However, the basement lacked windows, and the main level of the house—including the front door leading outside—could be accessed only by climbing a flight of stairs, which Dan, of course, couldn't negotiate. Not only did this set-up pose a threat in case of a fire or other emergency, but it was intensely restrictive. Dan had no independent access to the world beyond the basement walls; not only was he unable to leave the basement without help, but he couldn't even see outside—no grass, trees, flowers, birds, squirrels, or sunshine.

Dyke's and my last visit was disturbing. Because Dan had run into a doorway or some piece of furniture with his motorized wheelchair, possibly during an IED outburst, the wheelchair had been moved upstairs, to be used only when he left the house. Except for the occasional medical or dental appointment and Dave's visits, Dan sat on a couch in front of a TV all day. His only daily interactions were the moments when Audra or Marshall performed some chore for him, like helping him to the couch or bringing his meals, which he ate alone. In effect, Dan lived in solitary confinement.

During this period, I was scouring the internet and requesting recommendations from health care and social service professionals, seeking a facility specifically set up for TBI survivors, or at least a place geared toward younger, more active residents rather than the elderly clientele more typical of nursing homes. I wanted to find a collective residence where Dan might be able to live safely with others who shared his or similar problems, staffed by people who *understood* those problems—a place where he might find acceptance and maybe even companionship. It was heart-rending to know that I was likely hoping for too much. From both my internet explorations and the professionals I contacted, I learned that few such places exist anywhere in the United States. And for families who were not wealthy, there were precisely zero.

★ ★ ★

Fortunately, following Dan's move to Taylor Heights, Dave never did remove Dan's name from the waiting lists of long-term care facilities in the Atlanta area. As I was still seeking a place for him that would be less isolating and more accessible than Audra and Marshall's basement, Dave received a call from Trinity Village. There was a vacancy, and Dan could fill it if he wished. After his post-Taylor Heights experiences—his traumatic eviction from Carl's, then his basement confinement with Audra and Marshall—while Dan didn't exactly embrace the prospect of living in a nursing home, he was less resistant to it. Trinity Village had a good reputation, not only in online reports but also among the professionals Dave spoke with. Located in the Atlanta Metro area in Georgia, it was a long hour's drive from Dave's home—not rock-skipping distance, but not prohibitive for weekly visits, either.

So, in May 2006, Dan moved in.

5 Life at Trinity Village
2006–2017

Trinity Village is an impressive complex located on 500 wooded acres in Metro Atlanta. Despite its proximity to the megalopolis, its grounds are green and serene, fragrant with the omnipresent breath of sheltering pines and, in the spring and summer, vibrant with staccato birdsong. The campus is composed of an array of buildings devoted to distinct populations with specific needs. The Skilled Nursing and Rehabilitation Center is one of them.

Dan moved to Trinity Village in the spring of 2006. He expressed his sense of separation from those around him early on. Throughout the first weeks of our phone conversations, he spelled, "OLD AGED," "OLD TRINITY VILLAGE," "OLD HOME," and "ALONE ME." As he became more acclimated, however, he began taking part in facility activities, like weekly video movie screenings and occasional musical performances by local volunteers. The functions were geared toward his parents' generation—the movies were tame, and playlists for the musical presentations were dominated by hits from the 1930s and 1940s—but even if these activities weren't particularly engaging, they gave him something to do. He regularly attended resident gatherings even though his aphasia kept him from contributing anything more than his presence. And although Dan was agnostic, he attended church on the grounds every Sunday because it gave him somewhere to go and people to see. In other words, he did everything he could to become an active part of the community. It wasn't the community he would have chosen for himself—it was designed for his elders, not for him—but he did his best to participate in it, to optimize the circumstances in which he found himself. It didn't entirely relieve his existential loneliness and boredom, but it made them to some degree less oppressive.

It also helped that not everyone Dan encountered at Trinity Village was elderly. He actively enjoyed interacting with some of Trinity Village's staff members, most of whom were his own age or younger and

DOI: 10.4324/9781003340294-5

who gave him a sense of more "normal" social engagement. He carried on pleasant acquaintanceships with various physical therapists, CNAs, and nurses. A select few of these people Dan considered friends, and he learned their work schedules and looked forward to their shifts so that he could visit them. These associations were critically important to him. Given his aphasia, establishing and nurturing these relationships required more time, attention, and communicative ingenuity from both sides than most people are willing to invest, and these connections gave him a sense of normalcy. His friends were normal people who engaged in normal life, who liked him and treated him like the person he felt himself to be, which helped him to feel valued in an environment in which he otherwise (and increasingly) felt set aside. He finally felt a degree of belongingness.

Unfortunately, most job positions in nursing homes are filled by people whose future plans lie elsewhere. The work is often as poorly paid as it is demanding, so turnover rates tend to be high. Over time, Dan lost crucial friendships as staff members left, for reasons as diverse as returning to school, joining the military, getting married, relocating to other areas, and accepting better-paying, less grueling jobs elsewhere. Losing these relationships, some of which had developed over several years, was painful for Dan, leaving absence where presence had been. And for someone with aphasia, those empty spaces were not easily filled.

Countering the unpredictability of Dan's relationships at Trinity Village, Dave provided a source of steadfast love, friendship, and belongingness. Dan and Dave's outings—trips to Hooters or the Oasis (a local Atlanta strip club) for lunch, to the movies or the barber shop; occasional weekend afternoons or holiday celebrations at Dave's home with his family—formed the high points of his weeks. Reflections on the time Dan spent with Dave dominated our weekly phone conversations. In fact, Dan was my main source of Dave's family news—vacations he took; changes in his or his children's jobs, residences, or marital status; and the arrival of new grandchildren.

Besides the weekly visits and afternoons at his home, Dave occasionally took Dan on special extended weekend trips to the beach, the horse races, or overnighters at hotels for what Dan later termed "WILD PARTIES"—room service, porn movies, and now and then the attentions of a prostitute (when Dave gave Dan privacy by spending an hour in the hotel lounge). I confess to my own discomfort about lunches at strip clubs and hotel binges with porn and prostitutes, but if ever there were an argument to be made for the sex industry, for me this is it. Sex is not an existential need like air, food, or water, but it *is* a primal drive, as well as a heavily freighted realm of cultural importance, rife with signified meanings. Enabling Dan to experience himself as a sexual being, in a world in which he otherwise had virtually no chance to do so, was a gift of inestimable value. Not only did he enjoy the purely physical unleashing of sexual energy, but undoubtedly there were also psychosocial benefits that lasted much longer than the "wild parties" themselves. Paradoxically, perhaps, but nevertheless truly, these encounters and Dan's memories of them helped him to feel *normal*.

★ ★ ★

The contours of Dan's life at Trinity Village, as well as its underlying structure, were most fully sculpted by those charged with his daily care. I suspect, in light of the way events unfolded, that Dan's care providers were increasingly unable to relate to him, until their initial goal of addressing his needs was eclipsed over time by a new goal: controlling his behavior. This conversion began as early as 2006 and likely deepened with each IED episode. From the beginning, drugs were viewed as ammunition, the medium of a preemptive assault on Dan's rages. Three months after moving in, following a disruptive altercation with his roommate, Dan was relocated to a different room. On a phone call with me a month later, he reported that he was taking medication that made him feel "OLD," "SICK," "DIZZY," and "WEAK," and he was having difficulty moving his legs. It seems likely that, as long as he was kept in this condition, he was indeed less likely to react to IED triggers with intense outbursts, but he was also incapacitated and felt terrible. In a refrain that I would repeat several times over the next decade—and that I find deeply distressing in hindsight—I encouraged Dan to give his body time to adjust to the drug. I assumed that a new drug would only be prescribed for his benefit and that competent medical professionals would closely monitor him for side effects. In retrospect, these assumptions were ill-founded and naïve. On a call two weeks later, when he still wasn't feeling better, I offered to call the director of nursing to discuss the situation, but Dan asked me not to. Staff had made clear to him that taking the drug was a condition of his continued residence at Trinity Village. He feared eviction, in which case, he told me, he thought he'd be sent back to Audra and Marshall's house, or some similar situation. He was more troubled by the prospect of living in circumstances that might be as bad (or maybe even worse) than those he had just escaped than he was by the ill effects of the drug. With both of us still hoping the side effects would turn out to be temporary, he opted to ride them out.

Just over three and a half years elapsed before he again mentioned a bout of serious trouble. Dan has a heightened sensitivity to cold, and he and his roommate Frank frequently argued over the temperature of their room, which was chronically too chilly for Dan and too warm for Frank. In April of 2010, as they were scuffling for control of the thermostat, Frank lost his balance and fell on top of Dan. The nursing director blamed Dan alone for the altercation, I suspect because of his IED history and his inability to speak, to explain his view of the situation. He told me that she had threatened to press charges against him (as he understood it, to send him to "JAIL"), or, at a minimum, to kick him out of the facility. "SAVE ME," Dan spelled. I made a slew of phone calls, and Dave attended a facility hearing the following week. The matter was resolved—or at least it blew over—but the fracas doubtlessly generated another strike against Dan, both in his medical record and in his care providers' esteem for him.

Little more than a year later, in 2011, Dan answered the phone for one of our weekly calls from bed, after receiving an injection following another outburst. I don't know how often he was seized by IED episodes, since he only mentioned those whose effects overlapped with our phone calls, nor do I have more than circumstantial evidence of Trinity Village's strategy for dealing with them. At that point, though, it seemed that Dan was receiving medication episodically, on a perceived as-needed basis, while in the throes of explosive storms—unless such injections were given *in addition* to an ongoing drug regimen, which now seems possible, and perhaps likely. Because his IED bouts are transitory, usually lasting less than a minute or so (if properly responded to), giving Dan injections during or shortly following an episode would have been ineffective, except to the degree they served as punishment for a neurological disorder he couldn't control.

It's worth stressing here that, even throughout these years at Trinity Village, which were undeniably peppered with IED episodes, Dan was more than the sum of a series of neurological storms. He continued to strive to make the most of his life, and aside from his outbursts (which are admittedly unpleasant for everyone involved), he continued to exhibit the cheer, optimism, and ready sense of humor that have defined him within our family for his entire life. But finding even momentary contentment at Trinity Village was becoming increasingly difficult for him, as his relationships with personnel were progressively sullied, perhaps by a lack of understanding of IED or of strategies to defuse the outbursts, as well as by the unpleasant nature of the rages themselves. For at least some staff members, empathy for Dan, if it ever existed, waned with each episode. They saw him as ill-tempered, irrational, unpredictable, and intransigent. And he was well aware that he was neither liked nor respected, a circumstance that likely lowered the threshold required to trigger the storms, most likely increasing their frequency and intensity.

In 2012, Dan's life at Trinity Village reached a turning point. An IED storm at the end of May took Dan to the very edge of a chasm that marked an unscalable divide between him and the nursing home staff. Seven months later, in December, he tumbled over that edge and fell headlong into the abyss. Dan wasn't physically evicted from Trinity Village, but he apparently lost any toehold he'd ever had on belongingness with those around him, and he had little chance of acceptance even on the fringes of his community for the rest of his time as a resident.

★ ★ ★

Over the years, the pattern has become clear: Dan's IED episodes are aroused when his already chronically high levels of existential tension are coupled with the feeling that he is being underestimated, disrespected, or ignored, or when he feels thwarted in his continual efforts to determine the contours of his own life and shape its details. In an uninjured brain, neural circuitry established during maturation typically enables its bearer to contextualize and moderate troublesome feelings most (but by no means all) of the time. Like nearly all severe TBI survivors, Dan's neurological activity is disrupted, as DAI hampers communication within the brain itself. The apparent result is impaired mediation between Dan's emotions and his behavior, leading to more extreme reactions to his experience of anger.

Furthermore, the character of Dan's life circumstances provides innumerable triggers for anger. Like all of us, Dan wants to feel in control of his life, but both his impairments and the nature of life in a nursing home generate nearly continual reminders of dependency and powerlessness, and also subject him to the whims and timelines of others. And like most people in the United States, Dan grew up with the idea that independence and autonomy are essential markers of responsible adulthood—and, even more explicitly, of manhood. Although our cultural environment seems to be increasingly aware and more accepting of people with impairments, our late-twentieth-century upbringing immersed us—Dan, me, and most of the people whom Dan encounters in his everyday life—in messages that equate impairment with inadequacy and categorical inferiority.

This cultural messaging affects the way Dan sees himself. Even well-meaning people often inadvertently react to Dan with condescension, aversion, or complete dismissal. He is perfectly able to read the social cues that express these reactions. He understands them in part because he himself was acculturated to respond to impairment in the same way. His accident has certainly driven home the lesson that people with impairments are not necessarily lesser—that often, in fact, they have had to develop greater stores of courage and strength than most people, tempered by adversity. But I suspect that the aversive messages Dan internalized about impairment in his youth still haunt his psyche, usually humming in the background but brought vividly to the forefront when he feels denigrated. The complicated, uncomfortable, and often disheartening dance between what sociologist Erving Goffman calls "the normals" and "the stigmatized"[1] all too often validates Dan's suspicion that others tend to disregard or disrespect him. His own dependence on others—a condition he must face multiple times a day, as he waits on call lights to be answered, to be helped out of bed or into it to begin or end his day, to be showered and shaved, for food to arrive when he's hungry—sets the backdrop for feeling "lesser" that erupts into IED storms.

No doubt, Dan's constant struggle to view himself positively in the face of his impairments occasionally leads to an incorrect perception that he is being undervalued and disrespected. Justified or not, the perception itself is likely to provoke an IED episode, generating and fueling the proverbial "vicious cycle": Dan feels belittled or undermined, which elicits an IED storm, which leads others to regard (and treat) him as incompetent, immature, and socially unpleasant, which affirms his perception that he is viewed as inferior, which reinforces the thoughts and feelings that provoke IED behavior—and so on. Not incidentally, when Dan is viewed by others as incapable of conducting a positive, healthy relationship, his dependence on those others becomes even more evident (and more distressing) because of their avoidance or neglect. This dynamic, too, is self-feeding: the more Dan is reminded of his reliance on people he believes (accurately or not) don't like or respect him, the more frequent and intense his IED outbursts are likely to become, and the more definitively he is viewed as someone who isn't capable of forming or maintaining relationships—someone who doesn't belong within the community, and who therefore merits the avoidance and exclusion he receives.

★ ★ ★

In May of 2012, I received a call from Trinity Village staff informing me that Dan had tried to "run down" two CNAs with his motorized wheelchair and that his endangerment of personnel could not and would not be tolerated. I was horrified. Of course the facility could not allow Dan to harm others, I said, but knowing my brother as I do, I was confident that he would never intentionally hurt anyone. His outbursts were disagreeable and loud, sometimes even alarmingly so, but they were all sound and fury; even in the worst of them, he had never injured anyone. I promised to talk to him. I strive to be clear-eyed about my brother, and

I was ready to accept and deal with whatever had happened, but I also know there are typically at least two sides to every story. And I hadn't yet heard my brother's.

As soon as I hung up, I called Dan. He told me that he had indeed been upset, that his aggravation began early that morning when Opal, the CNA who was supposed to shave him, didn't show up. Nobody told him that she wasn't coming, no one arranged to shave him in her stead, and no one responded to his call light so that he could remind them that he had yet to be shaved. At length, he left his room and went outside to sunbathe, coming back onto his floor at noon to eat lunch in the dining room. After lunch, still wanting his shave, which was now five hours overdue, he returned to his room and again tried to attract a CNA's attention by using his call button. After half an hour, the light remained unanswered, and he wheeled down to the nurses' station. He was admittedly angry now; his repeated requests for help had gone unheeded, and he was now determined to be noticed. The nurses' desk was unattended, but he saw two staff members in one of several windowed cubicles behind it. He knew that these office and lounge areas were off-limits to residents. Nevertheless, he steamed past the desk and entered the cubicle to the women's consternation. They berated him, which added to his aggravation, triggering a full-blown IED storm that had been five hours in the making. Arms flailing, he accidentally knocked over a portable ice chest on a table by the doorway, scattering ice on the floor and alarming the two women, who felt trapped behind a desk in the small space, blocked from the entrance by Dan's wheelchair.

The chain of events seemed logical enough to me: Dan felt spurned when no one came to shave him or to offer any revised timeline or explanation for the oversight. He felt further slighted when his call light repeatedly went unheeded. For over five hours, no one had checked in with him, despite his sporadically repeated attempts to draw their attention. By the time he saw the two staff members clearly visible just beyond the unmanned nurses' station, and apparently available to help him but unwilling to so much as acknowledge him, he felt intentionally ignored—not important enough to justify consideration, deemed unworthy of even baseline concern. To him, it seemed he simply didn't matter to them. And I couldn't argue against that interpretation. His anger was as understandable as it should have been predictable, and he railed in his necessarily nonverbal, neurologically untempered way of asserting that he did, indeed, matter.

This dynamic was familiar, whether Trinity Village personnel recognized it or not: Dan had felt—justifiably, in my view—disregarded, and the result was an IED storm. The difference this time was that Dan had invaded an area deemed the sole province of staff. Dan's trespass into their "safe" space had made them feel unsafe.

I offered that viewpoint to Dan, which he understood and accepted as likely, and I promised to explain Dan's perspective to the CNAs. "Is there anything else you want me to tell them?" I asked.

"SORRY," he spelled.

"I'm so sorry that you couldn't tell them yourself," I said. "It's got to be hard not to be able to tell your side of the story, or even to apologize for getting upset."

"YYYYES," he typed, the extra Y's indicating the intensity of his frustration and exasperation.

After speaking with one of the offended parties, I called Dan back. "She said she forgives you," I told him. "Just don't scare people, okay?"

"FINE," he said.

But although the incident shifted from present alarm to past disturbance, it wasn't truly resolved. It lingered in perceptions and feelings about Dan. His trespass demonstrated that he had the ability to upset others' equilibrium. On that day, if not before, he had crossed categories, from episodically bothersome annoyance to potential threat.

★ ★ ★

Dan's trouble in May was followed by a rash of episodes that suggest a shift in the amount of concern and attention he received at Trinity Village. That summer, he had three serious falls that, in retrospect, suggest a likely alteration in his medication status—either the introduction of a new drug or an increased dosage of a drug (or drugs) he was already being given in an attempt to control his behavior—and a lack of monitoring or dosage adjustment for side effects. In June, on one of his outings with Dave, he fell in a public bathroom and badly bruised his back. The following month, he fell again, this time in his own bathroom at Trinity Village, and hit his head, requiring three stitches in an emergency room. In light of the June fall, I asked him following the July incident if he was having more trouble with his balance, and he replied, "MAYBE," and pledged to be more "CAREFUL." But in August he fell again. And I logged at the time that he was unusually difficult to understand on recent phone calls. I wonder now if, in that third fall, he sustained a concussion—more TBI—that affected his cognition, at least temporarily and possibly even long-term, or if some medication was compromising his ability to think and communicate. And I regretfully wish I had driven down to Trinity Village to speak with the nursing staff and administrators, not only to get a better sense of what was happening but also to demonstrate that Dan's family cared, and cared deeply, about his well-being.

Instead, I assumed at the time that these accidents were just unfortunate, unavoidable mishaps. I never thought to question whether or not Dan was receiving appropriate care. I'm wiser now and aware of the extent to which our culture encourages blind trust in the beneficence, capability, and authority of the people and institutions that tend us and our loved ones. Too many of us don't question treatment or conditions when warranted. I didn't. And that lack of questioning may have been interpreted as a lack of interest in Dan's well-being. One of the hard-learned lessons from my brother's experiences at Trinity Village is that constant vigilance, hands-on family engagement, and even forceful intervention when warranted are a vital part of ensuring the welfare of those who live in long-term care facilities. Because of the cultural authority these institutions are afforded, questioning their practices or actions may feel transgressive, like an overstepping of boundaries. But having failed to ask questions when questions were called for—that feels much worse.

I do believe that my reticence to question the beneficence, competence, and authority of personnel at Trinity Village paved the way to Dan's decline. Regretfully, I believe there's a direct line among Dan's decision, long in the making, in April of 2017 to stay permanently in bed, his near death seven months later as a result of sepsis and malnourishment, and the unrestrained hand Trinity Village exercised over him throughout at least the last five years of his life there.

★ ★ ★

Because of the incident in May 2012, when a CNA called me in December, nearly in tears, to tell me that Dan had "moved like he was going to run into" her in his wheelchair, I was already distraught when I phoned Dan. Not yet having heard of DAI or IED, I hollered, "You've got to stop that! You're going to get kicked out!" He hung up on me. When I called back half an hour later, I apologized, acknowledging that I should have asked him for his perspective instead of dressing him down, but I emphasized that I was as worried about what such actions might mean to his own well-being as I was about others' safety. Again, he assured me that, although he had been angry with the CNA, he never would have hurt her. "But *she* thought you were going to hurt her," I said. "Inflicting that kind of fear is, in itself, an attack of sorts. It does damage. I don't know what to do since you can't seem to control your outbursts, so I don't know how we're going to prevent this kind of trouble from happening again. But Trinity Village isn't going to keep letting this problem slide."

As it turned out, I was right. When I phoned Dan the next day, I was informed that he'd been taken to Cornerstone Hospital, a nearby psychiatric facility, for observation and assessment. I called the hospital immediately to talk to Dan, to reassure him that he wasn't alone, to let him know that I knew where he was, cared about what was happening, and would be keeping tabs on him. But I wasn't allowed to speak with him. Dave was listed as his primary contact, and Cornerstone would give Dan's patient ID number only to him. Because of privacy act restrictions, even Trinity Village couldn't relay the number to me, and without it, Cornerstone wouldn't even confirm to me that Dan was a patient there. I asked the receptionist to please tell Dan that his sister was trying to reach him and would talk with him as soon as possible. She said that if he were in fact there, she would relay the message.

Dave was out of town for the day and I couldn't reach him. I wasn't able to get Dan's ID number until the middle of the night, when Dave answered my host of frantic voicemail messages. I called Dan the next morning. Whether from anxiety and confusion or from some medication he'd been given, he was all but incoherent, and the conversation was relatively brief and wholly unsatisfactory, as I recorded in my phone log:

"Are you doing okay?"
"NO WEEK."
"You'll be there a week?"
"MAYBE."
"Are they doing tests?"
"NO."
"Is a doctor talking to you?"
"COLD FRE—"
"You're freezing? Are you chilly?"
"NO YES ROOM."
"Your room is cold?"
"TV NOWHERE WHEELCHAIR."
"I can call at nine tonight. Do you want me to?"
"NO MUSIC."

At this point, someone on Cornerstone's staff took the phone from Dan. "We need to use the phone now," she said, in a clipped tone.

"How's Dan doing?" I asked.

"Good."

Given the conversation we'd just had, that didn't seem likely. "Without a wheelchair, how's he getting to the bathroom?"

"We take him." The click of her tongue was only barely restrained.

"Would you please ask Dan if he wants me to call tonight at nine?"

She did and he said no. I thanked her and hung up.

Dan was at Cornerstone for a full week, from Monday to Monday. Our calls during that week were brief, mostly allowing us just to touch base. Our conversation on Sunday was a bit lengthier, more informative:

"HI," he spelled.

"Have they told you when you're going back to Trinity Village?"
"NO SIX DAYS."
"Yes—it's been six days, so I'm thinking maybe you'll be released tomorrow. What have you been doing at Cornerstone since you've been there?"
"DOCTOR."
"You've been talking to a doctor?"
"YES."
"Just once? Or more than once?"
"FIVE."
"You talked to him every day last week, then? Was he nice?"
"YES."
"Did he explain things to you—let you know what was going on?"
"NO."
"That's too bad—I'd like to know what's going on, and I bet you'd like to know too, wouldn't you?"
"YES DUMB ALL."
"They're all treating you like you're dumb? Is that what you're saying?"
"YES."
"I'm guessing they're kind to you; they just aren't treating you like an adult with his faculties."
"YES."
"If you don't go home tomorrow, I'll find someone to talk to and let them know they have to let you know what's going on. You shouldn't be kept in the dark. So when you told me you'd be going home over the weekend, you were just guessing?"
"YES."
"When's the last time you talked to Dave?"
"WEEK."
"You haven't talked to him since he left town?" Dave had flown to San Diego that Thursday to spend time with his older son Glen and Glen's young family, a Christmas holiday visit planned months in advance.
"YES NO."
"Didn't he see you on Wednesday before he left? I think he did."
"NO SUNDAY SIX DAYS NOW."
"So it's been a whole week since you talked to him? I'm surprised. You must have been feeling kind of stranded."
"YES."

I was shocked at the news that Dan had gone through this entire ordeal on his own, with only phone calls to remind him that he had family. How could I not have known? Why hadn't Dave and I collaborated? Why hadn't Dave acted? Why hadn't I?

Reasons are explanations, not excuses. There are reasons that explain situations, even when there are no excuses that justify them. In my case, I lived several states away. I had a more-than-full-time job. Visits to Atlanta were neither easy nor inexpensive. And Dave and I seldom spoke—not because of any intentional avoidance but because, since adulthood, we'd taken paths that didn't often cross. But this time, as a result, I didn't know how isolated Dan had been at Cornerstone. As for Dave, he was doubtlessly burned out, exhausted from putting out fires. He'd been a steady presence for Dan for years. No one had ever explained Dan's IED to anyone in our family. We had no name for it and no understanding of how little intention was involved, how commonly it attended TBI, or how essentially uncontrollable it was; we had only the experience of it. It seemed like willful behavior that continually caused trouble not only for Dan but also for Dave, and to a lesser extent me. Dan's move to Cornerstone was an escalation of trouble that was constantly on the horizon, breaking out with unpredictable frequency for years, but it was not a new problem. Dave's life, his experience, counted for something too. Between the two of us—Dave and me—I should have stepped in to fill the void during this period that undoubtedly had traumatized Dan. Both of my brothers had needed me to step up. But I hadn't, and the moment had already passed—Dan was returning to Trinity Village the following day.

"I should have come, Dan. I didn't realize you were all alone. I should have, though, and I'm really sorry. Dyke and I have plans to come visit you a week from Saturday to celebrate Christmas with you." It felt to me like too little, too late, but better than nothing, which is probably how it felt to Dan, too. I continued, "Have you been taking any medicine since you've been at Cornerstone?"

"YES."

"Is it medicine to calm you down?"

"YES."

"Does it seem helpful to you? Does it make you feel better?"

"MAYBE."

"You think maybe it helps you?"

"YES."

"That's good, anyway."

I wonder now if this was the moment Dan was put on Risperdal, and I wish I had asked the staff at either Cornerstone or Trinity Village for the name of the medication he was given, and then researched it myself. But I didn't. I trusted that medical personnel had Dan's best interests in mind—that this medication would circumvent his behavioral storms without causing him harm, and that he'd be monitored for negative side effects. Again, I was wrong.

"Well, I'll call you tomorrow. I think you'll be back at Trinity Village then, but I'll talk to you wherever you are."

Hindsight has a powerful capacity to generate remorse, to shame. Hindsight insists that I should have flown to Atlanta as soon as Dan was removed from Trinity Village. I should have arrived on Cornerstone Hospital's doorstep and done everything I could to ensure the emotional as well as physical well-being of my aphasic, hemiplegic brother. Hindsight drills down: my presence was called for—not so much to guide treatment (although maybe some of that too) as to provide Dan with belongingness through a presence that would demonstrate familial love and engagement, not only to Cornerstone and Trinity Village, but to Dan himself. I deeply regret, and wish I could change, not having offered my presence in this moment, as well as at other times when an act of solidarity would have made Dan feel less isolated, less at the mercy of a world that often must have felt merciless.

★ ★ ★

On Monday, December 17, 2012, Dan returned from Cornerstone Hospital to Trinity Village, but a lot had changed in his absence.

The two most obvious changes were that Dan was required to take a new daily medication, and he was no longer allowed to use his power wheelchair. Before leaving for a month-long vacation in New Zealand in mid-January, Dave secured a manual wheelchair for Dan, but he needed help to use it. Trinity Village staff complained that at times he was refusing medication, but he denied the charge, insisting that he was swallowing every pill brought to him. Despite following Trinity Village's orders, he wasn't consistently offered help with the manual wheelchair; consequently, he was spending nearly all of his days and nights sitting in his room when he wasn't in bed. He no longer had independent access to movie hours, resident newsletter meetings, roving visits with any staff that may have remained friendly, or church services. He had to rely on others to go anywhere, including to the bathroom, as he had at Audra and Marshall's. Dan was resigned to taking the mandatory drug even though it made him feel sick and weak, but this sudden confinement to his room was maddening.

While Dave was in New Zealand, Dyke and I visited Dan on alternate weekends. On one of these visits, I arranged to meet with Trinity Village's ombudsman, the liaison between facility administrators and residents and their family members. My daily phone calls to administrators, pleading for the return of a measure of Dan's independence, had been indulged but functionally dismissed—the administrators expressed sympathetic understanding, but nothing changed that would ameliorate Dan's misery. My meeting with the ombudsman, though, did seem to have some effect. As a compromise, she said, Dan would be permitted to use his power wheelchair. The speed regulator would be adjusted so that he could travel no faster than a slow crawl, and he could use the power chair only under staff supervision—which meant it would not be kept in his room.

On one of our phone conversations, Dan told me that no one had brought the chair to him a single time during the week, and he spelled "DIE."

"Are you saying you feel like dying?" I asked.

"YES," he answered.

In my phone log entry for this call, I wrote, "I left another voicemail for [the administrative director], this one stronger, saying that we need a pathway for Dan to get back in his chair." In a later phone call that same day, I asked Dan if he'd be interested in beginning physical therapy, noting in the log, "He needs things to look forward to. This is a very dismal period for him."

During a call later that week, Dan told me that he was missing Dave, that he continually felt like crying. "Clearly," I wrote, "Dave is Dan's lifeline. I'm helping, but he needs Dave around." In retrospect, while I'm sure that Dan did indeed miss his brother, I believe his spiraling loss of control over his life was the larger problem. A few days later, when he again reported that no one had been by with his wheelchair, leaving him to lie in bed, I was exasperated. "I just don't know what to do to light a fire under those people," I said. "I do think I've put you on their radar. Have you noticed a difference since I've been calling them all the time?"

"NO," Dan answered. "SUCK. MAYBE."

"You think maybe it would have been worse if I hadn't been calling so much?"

"YES," he spelled. "ALONE."

I reminded him again that Dave was returning in just a few days. But Dave's return was no panacea. Later that week, he took Dan on an outing to the barber shop and Hooters, and he told me afterward that Dan was alarmingly weak. Obviously, the medication and his forced confinement, along with the depression that his loss of autonomy had triggered, were taking a heavy toll.

The next day, the floor nurse called me, saying that Dan had declined lunch, refused to get out of bed, and spelled "DIE." She had requested an appointment for him with the staff psychologist but couldn't offer even an approximating guess at when he'd be seen. I told her that I believed Dan's root problem was being deprived of his power chair—effectively, of all independence, all self-direction, like when he'd lost his driver's license—and that I'd left a lengthy voicemail for the ombudsman just that morning. In the voicemail, I pointed out that Dan had been keeping his side of the deal but Trinity Village still wasn't giving him access to his power chair. As a result, he was diving into serious depression. The nurse promised to call the ombudsman too to add her own warnings to mine. There was at least one person at Trinity Village who cared, I thought with immense gratitude. Soon thereafter, I received a conference call from the administrative director, the director of nursing services, and the ombudsman. The consensus we reached was that Dan would be permitted unrestricted access to and unsupervised use of his power chair, as long as it was fitted with the speed governor.

Dan welcomed the news, but he was not as relieved as I had hoped he would be. "TWO MONTHS," he spelled. I thought at the time that he was lamenting his loss of two months of independence, and I emphasized that while we couldn't change the past, we would change the trajectory of the future. I believe now, however, that he was concerned that the previous two months of drugs and confinement had left him unable to take advantage of the measure of restored independence he was being offered. He spent the next few days in bed, muscles weak and trembling.

Over the following months, Dan began using his power chair sporadically, but its speed-governed sluggishness so frustrated him that, added to his weakened physical condition, he was increasingly reluctant to leave his room. A new medicine was added to his regimen, an appetite stimulant to combat his weight loss (at this point, only a pound), but he reported that it didn't make him hungry—only sleepy. By April, he was hardly using his Speak'n'Spell. Although we continued our phone calls, Dan relied to an ever greater degree on vocalizations to communicate; sounds of amusement or remonstration took the place of spelled words, and no longer did he inject topics or help guide conversations. Going back through the phone log entries for the summer, I noted that our discussions through this period were brief, with me pressing fruitlessly for responses. He wasn't unfriendly, and he still looked forward to my calls, but he apparently lacked either the ability or the motivation to spell with me. By November, I logged, "He didn't want to get the Speak'n'Spell out but was cheerily responsive to my blather." I summed up three weeks of calls in December prior to our Christmas visit with "He said nothing or practically nothing," and a few weeks later added, "I called—just didn't record it—just about all me talking these days. The tone of conversations is greatly changed; Dan just doesn't want to talk." It had been a full year since his traumatic admission to, and his equally traumatic return from,

Cornerstone Hospital—a full year of feeling mostly unwell and unhappy, his quintessential optimism increasingly dampened, as he became ever more resigned and disengaged.

And so his life went, for several years more. Finally, in April of 2017, Dan simply stopped getting out of bed.

★ ★ ★

There is consensus among scholars who study the phenomenon of belongingness that our need for belonging is likely an evolutionary adaptation, since the functions it performs increase the survival chances of individual social members (and therefore, macrocosmically, for the species as a whole).[2] We experience a lack of belongingness with the same intensity that we experience thirst or hunger, because when we are deprived of belonging, our chances of survival are diminished.

Overall, Dan's life at Trinity Village exemplifies that theory unfolding in real life. Aside from his family, Trinity Village constituted Dan's only possible source of belongingness. Over time, as a result of challenges to his social integration presented by the effects of TBI, not to mention the culture-wide, ineffable biases through which people with serious impairments are generally viewed, Dan was largely excluded from the baseline community acceptance that most of us take for granted. His inability to talk restricted his ability to negotiate either his self-presentation or his relationships, and the continual misunderstanding and underestimation that resulted from that constraint exacerbated both the frequency and the intensity of his IED episodes. The unfortunate complex of Dan's impairments, especially his neurological inability to prevent or explain his inevitable paroxysms of rage, pushed him continually further into social isolation. Others' inability to relate to him or to view him as an equally human being, with all the needs, feelings, and desires common to us all, severed even the most minimal ties of social obligation that belonging builds upon. In other words, Dan became a problem to be solved rather than a person to be cared about.

There was, too, a viciously cyclical aspect to Dan's life at Trinity Village. He experienced increasing levels of ostracism and rejection but was unable to do anything to lessen the growing gap between himself and others. As belongingness ebbed, what flowed in its wake was the pain and sense of impending doom that attend social disconnection, making him more susceptible to IED episodes, leading to further exclusion. As his ties to those charged with his well-being unraveled, protecting his dignity and personality (neither of which, I think, they believed in) became less important to them than ensuring his compliance.

Had Trinity Village personnel understood the differences between TBI and the conditions they were more familiar with (specifically dementia), would they have had more empathy for Dan and responded differently to his behavior? A more accurate and empathetic understanding of Dan and his neurological problems might have guided administrators and nursing staff to strategies that could have reduced the frequency and severity of his outbursts by helping him to feel more respected and cared about. Instead, he felt increasingly unmoored, and in turn defenseless and powerless, and then hurt and angry.

Dan has borne inestimable losses since his accident, but he has remained both capable and deserving of connection. Unfortunately, his impairments have too often been chalked up to temperament rather than neurology. At Trinity Village, he was variously regarded as hostile, obstinate, egocentric, irrational, or immature because of his brain injury. Although caring for him would have remained challenging and even unpleasant at times, informative training about the nature of TBI might have reduced the tension and resentment that had increasingly edged Dan out of belonging.

I believe that chemical restraint would never be considered acceptable treatment for anyone who is valued by those who conduct it. Once Dan had been functionally incapacitated with drugs, his life became increasingly sculpted by debility: a series of falls, persistent bed sores, dehydration, and chronic malnutrition, resulting at last in pain too severe to make getting out of bed worthwhile, and even an inability to shift his weight when he was in it. At that point, his near-fatal bout with sepsis (or something like it) was an almost predictable culmination of that chemical restraint. And so the last years of his eleven-year residence at Trinity Village graphically illustrate the theorized relationship between belonging and survival, in both psychosocial and physical terms.

I don't believe the social exclusion that led to Dan's suffering was necessarily intentional, or even conscious, but either way, the outcome was the same: his lack of belonging nearly killed him.

★ ★ ★

The question could very reasonably be asked—indeed, I have repeatedly asked it of myself over the past several years: when Dan began slipping, when he was finally unable to resist the near-total institutional domination of his body and his will through chemical debilitation and the imposition of rules that seized every vestige of his dignity and control over his life, why did I not step in? Why did I stand aside and allow his descent to go unchallenged? Why did I not fight for my brother?

In my own defense, I can answer only this: mine was not a failure of love—never of love—but of imagination. I failed to imagine better possibilities, a better life, for Dan. I lacked a model for what his life should (or even could) look like.

In part, my failure arose from a dearth of information. I had never heard of DAI, IED, or anosognosia until 2019, when I began researching medical literature for the purpose of writing this book. At the time of Dan's accident, the links between neurology, psychology, and behavior were not as well understood as they currently are (although there is still plenty of room for advancement in the field of neuropsychology). Medical professionals who spoke with my family offered little in terms of explaining the syndromes that are all but inevitable for most people with severe TBI. Survivors' difficulties were too overt to be unacknowledged, but health and care providers tended to view them as problems of damaged, diminished character, resulting from a newly aggressive egotism or the loss of logic, intelligence, or maturity. In fact, Dan's IED storms and anosognosic disconnections are purely organic, caused by disruptions in the transmission of neurological signals that are themselves the result of injuries to his brain, not of a flawed character. When Dan experiences an outburst, he isn't simply venting or "throwing a tantrum" or "acting out"; rather, in effect, his brain is short-circuiting. When he doesn't recognize the severity, or even the existence, of a specific impairment and therefore refuses to address or accommodate it, he is not being stubborn; he is neurologically unable to connect its practical relevance to himself or to his situation. Truly, the understanding that these issues are beyond his conscious control doesn't make them either more pleasant or more manageable, but—of critical importance—it does (or should) mitigate the anger and resentment that they can otherwise generate. Knowing that IED outbursts are the result of brain injury, and not of a nastiness that he is choosing to unleash, helps others keep their own inflamed emotions in check during Dan's rages, and to not hold him blameworthy afterward. As I have come to better understand the nature of his problems, I less often respond with anger, and I'm more often able to defuse situations. But even when I myself fly off the handle (as I sometimes do), once the storm is over, it's over as thoroughly for me as it is for Dan. That hasn't always been the case.

Tied into my previous lack of knowledge about the neurological effects of TBI was my culturally imbued, unquestioning adherence to the authority of medical institutions and nursing facilities, and my faith in the omniscience and benevolence of those who run and staff them. I had never heard of, and would never have imagined, the practice of chemical restraint before I confronted the issue firsthand, when my research triangulated Risperdal and Dan's misdiagnosis of schizophrenia with his increasing debility and unresponsiveness in communication. By that point, his will had been diminishing and his health had been declining for several years due to this form of behavioral control. That care providers might administer drugs that addled and immobilized those in their charge, and then fail to monitor for damaging and even life-threatening side effects, had been unthinkable—the premise of a bad movie, not the practice of a "skilled nursing facility." I had assumed that Dan's clear downward turn had been inevitable, the result of premature aging due to his various impairments, when in fact it had arisen from the mismanagement of his care by people who should have known better—who, in retrospect, didn't understand or were indifferent to my brother's well-being, who now appear to have been more interested in simplifying their workdays than in addressing Dan's psychosocial needs.

It wasn't until three months after Dan stopped getting out of bed that I began working to bring him to Indiana. The chain of events had been so improbable, yet so momentous: if Dave hadn't moved to Maryland, I wouldn't have begun the work to transfer Dan to another facility, and it seems likely that Dan's chemical restraint with Risperdal, as well as the bogus diagnosis of schizophrenia secured to justify it, never would have come to light. Dan would have continued to receive an antipsychotic that was destroying his body and ravaging his mind, shackling him to his bed, weak, dizzy, and trembling, and rendering him increasingly less able to communicate. As a result, his life had so diminished that he felt as though death would take nothing of value away from him.

I was unquestionably late to the scene—late in grasping the situation, its significance, its causes, and its stakes—but I had at last arrived. Dan deserved better, much better, than he'd been receiving at Trinity Village. And if he could survive long enough to get to Indiana, I would do everything in my power to make sure he got it.

Notes

1. Erving Goffman, *Stigma: Notes on the Management of Spoiled Identity* (Englewood Cliffs, NJ: Prentice-Hall, 1963).
2. Roy F. Baumeister and Mark R. Leary, "The Need to Belong: Desire for Interpersonal Attachments as a Fundamental Human Motivation" *Psychological Bulletin* 117, no. 3 (1995): 497–529. doi: 10.1037/0033-2909.117.3.497; Geoff MacDonald and Mark R. Leary, "Why Does Social Exclusion Hurt? The Relationship between Social and Physical Pain" *Psychological Bulletin* 131, no. 2 (2005): 202–23. doi: 10.1037/0033-2909.131.2.202; John T. Cacioppo and William Patrick, *Loneliness: Human Nature and the Need for Social Connection* (New York: W.W. Norton & Company, 2008); Kipling D. Williams, Joseph P. Forgas, and William von Hippel, *The Social Outcast: Ostracism, Social Exclusion, Rejection, and Bullying* (New York: Psychology Press, 2014); and Kelly-Ann Allen, *The Psychology of Belonging* (London: Routledge, Taylor & Francis Group, 2021).

6 Crossing the Rubicon

On November 26, 2017, Dan was discharged from Sugarbush Hospital having narrowly survived sepsis, with the hospital doctor recommending that he enter hospice. Instead, he returned to Trinity Village, still weak from his near-death battle, and still malnourished. The psychological re-evaluation required by Harbor Health, which had taken three months of effort and, finally, intervention by the State of Georgia to arrange, was scheduled for eight days later. I asked Dan if he wanted to postpone the appointment until he felt better, but he declined, and I was glad he did. I was confident that a fair appraisal of his mental condition, even in the immediate aftermath of traumatic illness and hospitalization, would affirm that he didn't have schizophrenia or schizoaffective disorder (or cerebral palsy!), and the sooner the record was corrected, the sooner he would be able to move to Indiana. The stakes couldn't have been higher: the results would determine the kind of facility that would, or would not, accept him.

Dan's appointment with Trinity Village's contracted psychiatrist was scheduled to take place in his room on Monday morning at 9:00, December 4. I flew down to Atlanta on Sunday afternoon and set up camp in a guest room three floors down from Dan's room. The accommodations were bare-bones (I knew to bring my own soap and shampoo), but clean and comfortable. Most importantly, I was near Dan. We spent an upbeat Sunday evening visiting. All Dan needed to do, I told him, was candidly answer whatever questions he was asked. Since candor is a hallmark of Dan's character, we both were optimistic that the evaluation would go smoothly.

After a surprisingly restful sleep, I went to Dan's room the next morning at 7:30. His breakfast tray was half an hour late, which made him nervous, not only because following established routines and knowing what to expect are particularly important to the equilibrium of TBI survivors but also because he wanted to be ready for the doctor. Still, once his meal arrived, he demonstrated a good appetite by dispatching a scrambled egg, a small heap of pulverized meat (neither of us could identify it, but probably bacon, sausage, or ham), and a slice of buttered toast.

After breakfast, I was surprised when Dan asked me to shave him. He was no longer scheduled for daily shaves, but he wanted to exude more polish for the psychiatrist who would evaluate his mental state. I had shaved him before, but always with an electric razor; I was wary of nicking him with his cartridge razor, and he laughed at my nervousness as I slowly, cautiously scraped his face with it. My efforts paid off: no blood, just smooth pink skin. Then, at his request, I dabbed his fresh face with Stetson cologne.

Following the shave, I was further astonished when Dan requested that I help him get out of bed and dress. Except for his trip to the hospital, he hadn't been out of bed—and he hadn't dressed at all—for eight months. He carefully picked out the clothes he wanted to wear, specifying even his nicest pair of underwear and newest socks. Because he hadn't been using his motorized wheelchair, it wasn't charged up and moveable, so I helped him into his manual wheelchair. However, the back angle of the chair was not adjustable, and he wanted to be able to see the doctor's face and meet his gaze when they met and when he answered questions. At my request, a CNA found a manual chair that tilted back, and Dan moved into it. He grabbed his brush and carefully groomed his hair.

At the end of the process, Dan was smooth-faced and fragrant, clothed in his finest jeans and t-shirt, and sitting up for the first time in months. My heart soared. I no longer felt as though I were pushing him, along with everyone else I was having to prod, to make the move to Indiana. His efforts demonstrated that he was an active partner in the enterprise. Although, throughout his life, my brother had defined himself (and been defined by others) by his exceptionally strong will, it was the first sign I'd seen in months of his desiring anything at all. I was thrilled by, and grateful for, his clear assertion of agency.

At 8:45, we were ready for the psychiatrist's arrival.

By 10:00, both Dan and I were getting agitated, although I tried to keep my anxiety to myself. My flight back to Indianapolis was scheduled for 2:00, which meant that I should be at the airport for check-in by at least 1:00. When booking my return flight, I thought I had given myself several hours of leeway. I checked with Trinity Village's staff, but they had received no word from the doctor about a delay, and efforts to obtain information from his office proved fruitless—no one knew quite where he was, nor could they contact him for an update on his schedule; he was simply out of the office, making his rounds.

By 11:00, I was insuppressibly unnerved. I went downstairs to the Director of Health's office in an effort to somehow salvage the situation. The psychiatrist didn't schedule specific appointment times for his visits, Paula explained, so he wasn't late. The 9:00 time I had been given was the earliest we could have expected him, not a firm hour for Dan's re-evaluation. Paula was sympathetic but at a loss for a remedy. The psychiatrist would get there when he got there.

As it turned out, the doctor arrived at noon. He'd moved Dan up in his schedule, he said, after receiving word from his office that we'd been expecting him earlier, and he was sorry for the miscommunication about appointment times that had caused such concern. The exam would be brief, he assured me, so I should have no problem catching my flight.

The evaluation was indeed brief—after three months of wrangling and supplication to the State of Georgia to get the appointment, it clocked in at about ten minutes. The questions seemed by turns vague, perfunctory, and obvious. The doctor began asking them in a tone appropriate for a preschooler, but as Dan answered them, with me interpreting his manual spelling, the tone shifted to one more befitting an adult conversation:

"Do you know what year it is?" (Dan offered the full date—month, day, and year—without being further prompted.)

"Do you know who's the current president?" ("DONALD TRUMP.")

"Do you sleep well?" (This question had a complex answer and so took a few minutes to convey: Dan usually has no trouble getting to sleep, but he often wakes up in the middle of the night, and occasionally he has trouble going back to sleep. "Like me," I observed, with a slight smile.)

"Do you ever hear voices or see things other people don't seem to hear or see?" ("NO.")

"Do you ever feel useless and hopeless? Do you ever feel that your life isn't worth much?" (Dan looked at me uncertainly. "ME NO." "Not to him," I told the doctor, who nodded as he recorded Dan's answer.)

"Do you think people talk about you and plot against you behind your back?" (Dan smiled uncomfortably at me with a small shrug and a nearly imperceptible nod. I expounded: "He's firmly grounded in reality, Doctor. He knows as well as I do that the staff at Trinity Village have repeatedly discussed him behind his back, and he also knows that some people have tried more than once to get him kicked out. There's nothing delusional about that." The psychiatrist nodded again, sagely making notations.)

After three months of finagling to get the re-evaluation, within ten minutes, Dan had passed with flying colors. "I can't remove the previous diagnosis," the doctor said, almost apologetically, "but I have recorded that he has no signs or symptoms of schizophrenia at this time, and I have changed the diagnosis of 'schizoaffective disorder' to 'TBI-associated mood disorder.'"

"That's all we were hoping for," I said, grinning, as I reached for and shook the doctor's hand. "Thank you."

Unfortunately, although he said a cordial goodbye to me, the psychiatrist left the room without so much as a parting glance at Dan.

Shortly after the doctor left, a CNA entered Dan's room with a clipboard, reading through a form that asked for Dan's preferences for various foods and activities. I was at this point pressed for time to make my flight, but Dan (and I, as his interpreter) answered each question thoughtfully. It seemed strange that, more than eleven years after he'd moved into Trinity Village, they would suddenly be asking him to clarify his likes and dislikes, now that we were in the process of arranging for his relocation to another state.

Once we were alone, I leaned into Dan for a tight hug. We beamed at each other. "I'm incredibly proud of you, Dan," I said. "The whole morning was so stressful—I was on the verge of losing my cool myself—but you managed to keep yours. I can't tell you how important that was, or how happy that makes me." I needed to express it, and I think it was good for him to hear, but even as I raced from his room to grab my bag and whisk away to the airport, he already knew.

We'd done it.

★ ★ ★

Harbor held its annual Christmas dinner for residents and their families on December 23, and Shiloh sent an invitation to Dyke and me. The event was spread over three consecutive evenings to limit attendance on any given night, resulting in not only a logistically more manageable enterprise for staff but also a cozier, more intimate experience for attendees. Dyke pointed to the invitation as a good sign: Shiloh, it seemed to him, viewed us as a prospective part of the community. I hoped he was right, but I also considered the possibility that we'd been invited simply because Shiloh and I had formed a friendly relationship over the previous four months, as she offered advice on how to find decent alternative places for Dan. While she had agreed to review documentation from his re-evaluation at Trinity Village, I was hopeful but not confident that the revision to his record would result in his acceptance at Harbor.

The facility sparkled with evergreen wreaths, clusters of gleaming glass bulbs, tinseled garlands, and half a dozen or so spangled Christmas trees bedecking various hallways and corners. Dyke and I were escorted to a low-lit dining hall set up with six or seven tables draped with red and green linens, with centerpieces of pinecones and ornaments. A middle-aged man sat alone at a small table in a corner of the room, alternately singing and playing a tenor saxophone as he performed karaoke to Christmas CDs. Residents and their families, some especially festive in sequined Christmas sweaters and Santa hats, chattered as they ate at their tables, pausing occasionally to applaud the entertainer. Dyke and I ate our vegetarian meals—salads, green beans and corn, dinner rolls, and slices of pie and ice cream—in good spirits. The food was standard institutional fare, but the ambiance was festive. And, we hoped, auspicious.

After the meal, Shiloh greeted us at our table and offered us a tour of the building. I had seen the entire facility in August, but Dyke hadn't, so we walked along the warmly lit hallways and ducked into unoccupied rooms. Dyke was as impressed as I had been on my first tour—by Shiloh and the staff as much as by the sparkling clean facility—but I was experiencing substantial bittersweetness. I sensed that Dan could have a real home here, a real life, but I didn't know if he'd get the chance to build it. More than ever, I wanted to bring him to this place.

★ ★ ★

Several weeks later, Dyke and I were eating pizza with Dyke's son in Chicago when I received an email from Shiloh, noting that she had received and reviewed updated documentation from Trinity Village. More records were still needed, she said, but she was confident that there would be no dealbreakers: "At this time," she wrote, "I have authorized the admissions team to start the transfer process. As soon as we receive the remainder of the paperwork from Trinity Village, we will start the request for transfer to Indiana!"

I didn't make a scene whooping and hollering in the pizzeria, but only because I exercised immense self-control. I was almost dizzy with joy and relief. The previous five months had seemed less like a roller coaster than a Tilt-a-Whirl—ups and downs augmented by unpredicted spins and pivots: revelations of false diagnoses and chemical restraint, Dan's brush with death by sepsis in the hospital, and the wrestling required to obtain his psychological re-evaluation. Finally—finally!—with one brief email, it seemed like the pieces were sifting seamlessly into place.

That weekend, Dyke and I drove down to Trinity Village to visit Dan. We were all upbeat—relieved and excited—despite the slight current of anxiety generated by the enormity of our shared undertaking. When we were leaving to return to Indiana, I told Dan, "The next time we come down here, it'll be to move you up to Muncie!"

Dan crossed his middle finger over his index finger.

"R," I began spelling.

He shook his head. He wasn't signing the manual alphabet. He was crossing his fingers to signify *hope*.

★ ★ ★

A week later, I wrote this entry in my journal:

> I got a call from Dave, who was worried about Dan, who had refused to take his prescribed blood pressure medicine, stool softener, and nutritional supplement shake. Dave had tried to convince Dan to stop being "resistant"—a word that seems to follow Dan around. Dyke was upset at the news on my behalf. Oddly, I wasn't upset at all—concerned, yes, but suspending judgment until I could talk to Dan.

I called Dan and asked him if it were true that he had declined the meds and the shake: "YES."

I asked him if he didn't want to drink the shake because he didn't like the flavor: "YES."

I asked him if he didn't want the stool softener because he had to use a bedpan and didn't like that: "YES." I stressed that eliminating toxins from our bodies is nothing to be embarrassed about—everyone does it, and everyone *has* to do it—and that if he wanted to work on using a toilet when he got to Muncie, he could, but in the meantime, he needed to get rid of his body's waste. I reminded him that the condition he'd almost died from in November likely had started with chronic constipation.

I asked him if he was worried about Trinity Village giving him medicine that he didn't need, or that otherwise wasn't good for him, as had happened with the Risperdal: "YES." I told him that the blood pressure medicine was necessary because he spent all his time in bed now, and, again, if he wanted to work on that in Muncie, Harbor would help, but in the meantime, he needed to maintain his health by taking the medicine. I promised him that I would carefully keep track of any meds he was given and that I would never allow what happened with the Risperdal to happen again—he wouldn't be asked to take any unnecessary medicines or any substance that would do him harm.

I reminded him that Dave and I almost lost our brother in the hospital two months earlier, and that's why we react the way we do when we think he's making a decision that jeopardizes his health and even his life. I asked him to think about these things, and I would call him back after ten minutes, and he could give me his answer then. "NO"—in effect, he didn't need to think about it; he already knew his answer. Was he going to take the medicine? "NO." I told him that it was indeed his right to make that decision, but that if he declined, I doubted Harbor would admit him into its facility: "Why would they bring you in just so you can refuse treatments you need and then die under their care?" I told him I'd call back in ten minutes for his answer and hung up.

I did call back, and he said he'd follow the doctor's orders. I clarified: the nutritional shake, the stool softener, and the blood pressure medicine? "YES." I thanked him for making that decision, told him I thought it was the best decision to make, and said I'd call him back for our reading session fifteen minutes later, at 10:00 (our usual time). I called the nurse's station and asked them to please give him the shake and medicines before 10:00. When I called at 10:00, he had already taken everything and was ready for our book.

Far from worrying me, this incident increased my confidence that Dan was going to do well in Muncie. We would work together by eliminating, to the greatest extent possible, dysfunctional patterns that had developed over years. I didn't want to pressure him into making the decisions I *knew* were right. Instead, I silently pledged that I would make an effort first to understand his objections, and so avoid blindly labeling (if only to myself) the behavior that stemmed from them as dogged, irrational "resistance." For years I had been arguing that Dan had, overall, retained his capacity for logical functioning. (While I hadn't yet encountered the terms *intermittent explosive disorder* or *anosognosia*, I *had* noticed that his bouts with illogic and spontaneous outbursts of anger consistently arose when others' perception of his capabilities conflicted with his own sense of them; in other spheres, his reasoning has remained reliably sensible.) I vowed to have faith in my own time-tested assessment of Dan's rationality and interact with him accordingly—work to understand his perspectives, lay out my own when they contrasted with his, help him to see angles he may not have considered, and take seriously whatever angles he might present that perhaps I had missed. And I would respect, to the best of my ability and with as much grace as I could summon, his right to be the final arbiter in any decisions about his own life.

In other words, I would take him seriously—as my brother, my equal, and my partner in the Muncie enterprise, but also as the agent who is responsible for making the decisions that compose the experiences of his life.

★ ★ ★

Dan's official acceptance at Harbor came through on February 5, 2018. Shiloh wrote, "I have a great room ready for Dan!" and sent photos: the room was clean and bright, the long wall a deep coral with facing walls a warm cream. Winter sunlight streamed through a window that opened onto a courtyard. A shallow alcove in front of the window added architectural interest and some extra space, premium features in any long-term care facility. The only furniture on his side of the room was a bed and two small, matching dressers in a light walnut finish, which added to the sense of spaciousness. Dan's room at Trinity Village, continually in shadow lessened only by artificial light, with its dingy cinderblock walls and battered wardrobe and chest of drawers, seemed dungeon-like by comparison. Harbor and Trinity Village were both nursing homes, but the difference between the room Dan currently called home and the room he'd soon be moving into could not have been more dramatic. The contrasting rooms dovetailed the contrast that I hoped Dan would find between his years at Trinity Village and a new life at Harbor, a life that was fresh, light, saturated with color, and rife with new possibilities.

I had already researched medical transport companies to find a service that would transfer Dan from Trinity Village to Harbor. I explored websites and sent exploratory emails before making a choice. The service I selected, based on its website and on email communication with the owner, sounded ideal. Of key importance, I could accompany Dan on the trip. Also, according to the website, the service was bonded and accredited, and its two-person transport teams passed rigorous background checks and included at least one EMT. Its specially outfitted, well-maintained fleet of "new comfortable transport vehicles" were equipped with stretchers overlaid with adjustable waffle mattresses for extra comfort. Additionally, the owner noted, all vehicles offered "separate rear air conditioning temperature controls, complimentary limited Wi-Fi internet service, AC electrical outlets capable of charging small electronics, Sirius XM Radio, and flat panel roof mounted DVD players for both the additional rider and passenger." Food and beverages would be provided for both Dan and me "according to dietary needs and restrictions through various methods, including restaurants." I was assured in the owner's email that "Our transport teams utilize empathetic bedside manners to ensure that your loved one is treated in the same manner that our team members would treat their own family members." In short, everything I was seeking.

With Dan's and Dave's approval, I booked the service for Saturday, February 17. Dave boxed up most of Dan's belongings the weekend before. Dyke and I would leave Indiana for Trinity Village on Friday morning; that night and the next morning we'd pack up anything Dave hadn't, and then Dan and I would make the trip to Muncie in the transport van. Dyke would follow the van in our car, loaded with Dan's belongings, and we'd arrive together that night at Harbor. This schedule left Sunday free so that I could help Dan feel more settled in his new home before I returned to work on Monday.

In preparation, I told Dan we'd have a "van party" on the ten-hour trip to Muncie, and I tried to make it festive. I bought a variety of Clif meal bars, several York Peppermint Patties, and a bag of Pepperidge Farm Goldfish Crackers in case he got hungry between restaurant stops, as well as a barrel of wipes for post-snack cleanups. I would take my iPad so that we could use the van's wi-fi to stream several horse-themed movies I had placed in queue on Netflix. We could also read from the book we were currently absorbed in, *The Horsemen: Inside Thoroughbred Racing as Never Told Before*, by Jack Engelhard. I was looking forward to a day of happy adventure to kick off this new chapter of Dan's life. But most of all, with a surging stream of optimism-infused determination, I was looking forward to Dan's new life in Muncie.

★ ★ ★

Friday evening, February 16, Dyke and I arrived at Trinity Village. Dyke worked on the packing while I began slathering Dan's Five Guys cheeseburger with ketchup for his dinner. Dan suddenly went motionless and his eyes widened. "REAL," he spelled. It took me a moment to understand that he was noting the first instant that he was experiencing the move from Georgia to Indiana as real—that it was actually going to happen. He crossed his fingers, and this time I recognized the sign, not as the letter "R" of the manual alphabet, but as an expression of hope. I promised him that his hope was warranted, that this move would improve his life.

As Dyke and I were leaving for the night with nearly everything jammed into our car, Dan scanned his empty room and again spelled "REAL." "The next time we see you," I said, "it'll be to move you to Indiana." Joy flooded his face and he put his hand to his forehead, eyes closed, as if to hold in the moment. He fairly glowed.

The next morning, Dyke and I arrived just after Dan finished breakfast. We collected toiletries and any remaining stray odds and ends that had escaped the previous night's packing and waited anxiously for the medical transport team to arrive. At 8:55—five minutes early—Marty and Jerry swooped into Dan's room, we signed the requisite paperwork, and they briskly lifted Dan onto the gurney, Jerry exclaiming, "He's light as a feather!"

Dyke and I trotted alongside the stretcher, making small talk with Jerry and Marty as they wheeled Dan down the hallway and into the elevator. After breezing through the lobby and its glass doors into the brisk February morning air, we paused as the team unlocked the van. "Say goodbye to this place, Dan," I said. "You won't be seeing it again." Dan pumped his fist into the air, then, laughing, raised his middle finger. Over the years, he had liked some of the people who worked at Trinity Village, but for the most part, especially in recent years, he had been miserable there, and he was thrilled to be leaving. Dyke told me later that he caught Dan's expression as we exited the lobby doors, and he recognized it as the same expression I had described to him in our motel room the night before: the look of a falsely imprisoned man at the moment of his vindication, realizing his freedom has been restored. It was, Dyke agreed, a look of sheer joy.

★ ★ ★

The trip from Union City to Muncie was not the party I had envisioned and promoted to Dan. First, of the two passenger seats I could choose from, one was placed several feet behind his head, and the other was down by his calves. Either placement interfered with our plans to watch movies together. Second, the van's wi-fi was out of commission, so we had no internet for streaming movies on my iPad. Instead, he watched videos by himself on my iPhone for as long as its battery lasted—the AC electrical outlets in the back of the van didn't work either, so I couldn't recharge my phone and had to keep some juice in reserve to coordinate with Dyke, who followed the van in our car. At least, that had been the plan. As Jerry cut through the heavy Atlanta interstate traffic, I glanced up at the speedometer to see that we were whizzing along at 110 mph. Dyke lost sight of the van almost immediately.

Still, maybe the trip wasn't too bad for Dan; he watched a documentary on the Kentucky Derby, we read a few chapters of the Englehard book, he watched a film about Bill Shoemaker, and then I read to him some more. In between we chatted, at one point rehashing old memories from our childhood years in Florida and Georgia.

Several hours into the trip, we stopped at a McDonald's. Dan waited on the gurney in the van while I went to the restroom, and Marty ordered a milk, a double cheeseburger, and a small order of fries for Dan. The stop took about ten minutes, and we were back on the road again. I helped Dan with his burger, fries, and milk, and, vegetarian that I am, I ate a blueberry Clif bar.

At one point late in the afternoon, Dan handed me my phone and signaled that he wanted a bit of silence. He looked up at the ceiling, his face a study of anxiety. He knew the life he was leaving had been hellish, but he had no real confidence in the kind of life he'd be entering. I had promised him it would be "better," but what, exactly, did that mean? Hadn't I had led him to expect a better trip than we were having? The van was noisy, the wi-fi and device-charging outlets didn't work, the meals weren't exactly stellar, and despite our whizzing speed, the ten hours were dragging by almost preternaturally slowly. Why should he believe in the rosy portrait I'd painted of life at Harbor? And for all I could tell, maybe I *was* leading him into disappointment. How could either of us be certain? I had done my homework before selecting Harbor, but I had also done my homework before selecting the transport company. What could I, and what couldn't I, predict—much less control?

I could predict (and control) only one thing: I would do everything in my power to ensure that Dan's life was the best I could make it. There were aspects of his experience I had never been, and never would be, able to control. I would try to manage whatever fallout might arise to whatever degree I was able, so that Dan suffered as little as possible and enjoyed as much as he could. I had to acknowledge that I couldn't guarantee a smooth road. I could inflate tires and patch potholes, but the road would doubtlessly be bumpy at times. Still, isn't that true for all of us? I would share his problems, shoulder some of the burdens, help in the ways that I could, and commiserate when he was troubled.

In retrospect, it was largely my inability to "fix" Dan's problems that had caused me to withdraw from his life forty years earlier following his accident. Driving the interstate between Fresno and Fullerton each weekend, tears coursing my cheeks both on the way down and then on the return trip, searching gift shops and card stores for the magic t-shirt or poster that would cheer Dan and help him regain what he'd lost, watching his eyes squint in pain or water with frustration, averting my gaze from the mix of food and saliva that dropped from his mouth as he ate or from the spreading stain on his pants that was emblematic of his loss of control—I shrank from the pain, leaving him (and the rest of my family) to deal with the problems without me. For six months following Dan's accident, I woke up every morning steeped in grief. I withdrew from the three evening classes I was taking at UC Fresno because I simply couldn't think. Weeping, I drank myself sick nearly every night, trying to banish the sense that life had betrayed us all. Finally, in May, I escaped by joining the Navy, letting it whisk me into a completely different life. I was absorbed in boot camp and C school and overseas duty stations as I put distance between Dan's new reality and mine. I abdicated my responsibilities as his sister, as my parents' daughter, as Dave's sister, because I was unable to solve his problems or assuage the seemingly unendurable pain he had been left with.

What I hadn't understood then, but was working hard to apply now, was that my job had never been to erase Dan's problems or his pain, but to help him bear them by sharing in his life. In his new life in Muncie, I would try to foresee and prevent problems and address those that arose, but I was neither omniscient nor omnipotent. While my best efforts hadn't sufficed in making the trip to Indiana festive, or even marginally pleasant, I could and would sit beside him, sharing the noise and the discomfort, showing him that he wasn't alone. And, following ten hours of unpleasantness, we did arrive in Muncie intact.

I had finally realized, and accepted, that I couldn't give Dan a smooth ride—then, now, or ever. The most important gift I could give him is belongingness, which I could only bestow through my presence. He belonged to me, and I belonged to him. All else would be gravy.

7 New Normal

After an exhausting day on the road, the medical transport van pulled into Harbor Health Care in Muncie, Indiana, at 7:30 on the evening of February 17, 2018. Staff had been alerted to expect us, and the admissions coordinator greeted us with a welcoming smile and a sheaf of admissions paperwork. Her manner was pitch perfect; she treated Dan with warmth, courtesy, and sincere patience. She explained each form, and I held the clipboard as Dan signed them all.

The first paper established his "code" status, referencing the DNR order he'd signed at Sugarbush Hospital in November. Did he still want to withhold intervention if he stopped breathing or if his heart stopped beating? He shook his head no, and I sought clarification: "You would want measures taken to save your life, is that right?" He nodded, and I silently rejoiced.

While Dan was painstakingly executing his fourth or fifth signature, I made an obliquely apologetic reference to our tiring day, hoping to account for how long the process was taking. The coordinator breezily waved away my comment. "He's doing great," she said. "I wish we didn't have to subject him to all this paperwork after the day he's had." That was how I felt too, but I was relieved and cheered to hear someone else say it, and I knew Dan was, too.

Once the admissions process was complete, we went to Dan's new room, where he was lifted into bed. I turned my attention to his dinner. Following the quick trip into McDonald's early in the afternoon, the only other stop we'd made was at a secluded rural gas station, and nothing in the convenience store would have appealed to Dan (or me). He ate part of an Oatmeal Walnut Clif bar and a Peppermint Patty, and I promised him dinner once we arrived at Harbor. Unfortunately, Harbor's kitchen had already closed. While Dan and I chatted, Dyke made a run to Wendy's for a double cheeseburger, a side salad with ranch dressing, and a chocolate frosty, and he picked up a bottle of milk at Walgreens. Not the healthiest

DOI: 10.4324/9781003340294-7

of meals, but Dan dispatched it with gusto. I took his healthy appetite as a good sign.

With the boxes of his belongings stacked in his room and Dan comfortably ensconced in bed, Dyke and I drove the fifty minutes to our home in Fishers. I would come back the next morning to help him begin settling in, but for the moment, Dan's situation seemed as close to perfect as I could have hoped for. Surfacing from our goodnight hug, he'd looked tired but relaxed and happy. The afternoon's anxiety, for both of us, had vanished. I thought, We're all going to sleep well tonight.

And we did.

★ ★ ★

On my way to Dan's room the next morning, I approached the hall's day nurse, Marjorie, for an update. "Everything going okay?" I asked, hopeful but not confident.

"Just fine!" Marjorie answered. She then showed me a chart of the manual alphabet that she had just finished laminating so that Dan could better communicate with staff. It would also help those who worked with him to learn to read his spelling fingers, she said. In my journal, I wrote, "Such a simple thing—why had no one (including me) ever thought of it before? He's in the right place."

When I went into his room, Dan was clean, well-rested, and cheerful. He conveyed that, so far at least, everything was going well. He'd already had a shower. He'd also received his initial weigh-in, and his eyes sparked fire when he told me that the scales had registered 108 pounds. "FIVE ELEVEN!" he signed, then clenched his fist. Before his accident, he had measured 5'11" tall, but his stint at Trinity Village had left him well under the official jockey weight that, as a lean and healthy adolescent, he had struggled but failed to retain as he continued to grow. Even worse, I thought to myself, that 108 pounds likely represented more than two months of weight gain, since Sugarbush Hospital's diagnosis of malnutrition in November had surely spurred Trinity Village to pay more attention to his eating. At the very least, they'd added supplemental shakes to his diet.

The weigh-in put an assessable number to the fragile state of Dan's health. I asked him if he thought that his overall physical condition might explain why getting out of bed had become too much for him the previous April—that the pain he experienced ("SORE") was caused by malnutrition. He nodded. If he could regain his strength, build up his muscles again, and feel better and more energetic from eating right and working on physical therapy, I suggested, maybe he'd want to move out of bed.

I assured him that, as we'd agreed in August, staying in bed for the rest of his life was a choice that he was completely free to make, but I also pointed out that if he made that choice, his life would almost certainly be shortened by years. He nodded agreement. I said that it seemed to me that he'd been viewing his life as not really much worth living, that at Trinity Village he'd ceased to experience enough pleasure or promise to justify the effort required to endure each day. He nodded gravely. I told him I understood—that for years he'd been treated like a naughty, ill-behaved toddler instead of like the man he is, and that his angry episodes had often been triggered by that treatment. He nodded, eyes widened in apparent surprise that I had connected those dots. I pointed out that he was only fifty-seven years old—that he still had years of living left, and that he could enjoy them. I mentioned the "Wall of Heroes" that celebrated Harbor's physical therapy successes. I affirmed that Harbor was a different kind of place from Trinity Village—that the people here would really care about him, that even before his arrival they'd been viewing him as a valuable person and would work hard to help him regain a real life—that enjoying his life was still possible, and that was precisely why I had worked so hard to get him into *this* specific place. I told him that Dave loves him as much as he loves his own life, and he'd repeatedly proven that he'd do anything he could for his brother and that I'd never say a critical thing about his love, devotion, or effort. But, I observed, Dave has a "buck up, suck it up" attitude, believing that whatever our circumstances, our job is to deal with them, to simply endure and outlast the hardship. Dan nodded somberly, again a bit startled that I was giving voice to his own understanding of the situation. I told him that I love and respect Dave with all my heart, but that I have a different philosophy—that I agreed with Angela Davis when she said, "I will no longer accept the things I cannot change; I will change the things I cannot accept." I repeated the quotation slowly, twice, and then asked, "Would you like to get out of bed again? Do you want to do more than lie in bed watching TV, waiting to die?" Firmly, deliberately, he nodded.

On my way out to the parking lot, I relayed Dan's decision to Marjorie, who received the news with a smile and a nod. "I was hoping for that," she said.

"Me too," I answered, gladness glowing in my bones.

★ ★ ★

The first weeks and months of Dan's residence at Harbor were marked by a flurry of activity. I visited Dan every day. Together we went through the boxes of his possessions, arranging what he wanted to keep and discarding the rest. His material attachments were limited: his entire household effects were a large-screen TV, a bag of clothes and toiletries, some framed family photos, a wall calendar, a globe, a large-print dictionary, and a fine heavy bronze statuette of a jockey on a racehorse in mid-stride. Most of his clothes were shabby, and he wasn't sure which actually belonged to him and which had been misdelivered by Trinity Village's laundry personnel; clothing circulated freely there, without much apparent concern for which resident was its rightful owner, and he had long since ceased to pay attention to which clothing was his. Soon after his arrival at Harbor, we replaced the ragged shirts and pants with new jeans, t-shirts in zippy patterns and colors, splashy new boxer shorts, and a dozen pairs of bright white socks. When I arrived for visits after work, Dan would be watching TV from his chair, clean-shaven and nicely dressed, hair neatly clipped and brushed.

Upgrading Dan's wardrobe was important for several reasons. First, it contributed to his sense that moving to Harbor signaled a new, better chapter in his life. When he got up in the mornings, he wasn't dressing in a stranger's threadbare clothing; he donned his own clothes, fresh and whole. Dan wasn't much interested in fashion trends, but his self-image was improved by knowing that he was respectably dressed and well-groomed. Also, he knew that these new clothes reflected my concern for him; they were a tangible sign of our connection. Finally, the revamped image Dan was now presenting served as a visible marker to others that he was a respectable man tightly enmeshed in a family that valued him. It reinforced the tacit claim that he was worth caring about, not only by his family but also by the people at Harbor and in the broader community—that he deserved acceptance and belonging.

That claim was one I was making, not Dan. He, like most of us, didn't explicitly think in those terms, and yet he had endured great misery resulting from a lack of belonging at Trinity Village. In the process of earning my doctorate in communication studies, I learned the various ways we communicate as well as the personal and cultural implications of the messages we send. I had a heightened awareness of the importance of belonging and the many ways we obtain, or fail to obtain, acceptance through communication. Nonverbal messaging always figures into how others view us, but because Dan's verbal communication is so compromised by aphasia, his nonverbal communication—with self-presentation serving as a chief component—is all the more pivotal in shaping the attitudes others form about him. And nonverbal communication includes more than facial expressions and gestures. Personal appearance is an indicator that others use to assess our place within the social world. The material possessions we surround ourselves with is another. We use multiple forms of nonverbal as well as verbal evidence to influence the quality, depth, and breadth of our social connections to others.

As a result of that dynamic, one of the most important actions I was able to undertake on Dan's behalf in the early months following his move was simply showing up every day. Daily visits accomplished a number of important ends. First and foremost, I was able to be of practical use to my brother as I served as his liaison with Harbor staff. Because he couldn't speak, he couldn't weigh in on schedules and preferences, but I could; he couldn't raise and work through misunderstandings and problems, but I could; he couldn't explain his perspectives, but I could. These pragmatic benefits of my daily presence were supplemented by less tangible ones. Demonstrating my commitment to Dan made the implicit assertion that he deserved belonging. Personnel could see that my interactions with Dan are "normal," proving that he is capable of participating in healthy, mutually pleasurable relationships. Also, when Dan and I experienced conflict, which we occasionally did, we were able to model his ability to perform his part in reconciliation. Finally, my frequent appearances helped me become part of Harbor's community too, which was of no small importance. As someone within the Harbor community, I could address problems differently than I could have as an outsider, as an occasional visitor. I proved my reliable sense of goodwill and solidarity with the facility's staff as well as with my brother. I considered us all—Dan, staff, and me—a team working for the same goal: everybody wins. I always advocated for Dan, but I worked hard to resolve any conflicts between his needs and those of personnel before pressing for any resolution.

Dan's continued bursts of IED presented an acid threat to the kinds of affiliation I was hoping to help him foster. Almost all the time, Dan was cheerful, cooperative, funny—in short, pleasant company, easy to like. But his periodic outbursts of rage injected a seriously negative element into the pursuit of the social and emotional belonging for Dan that I was aiming for. It takes only a few moments of sporadic over-the-top hollering, frenzied arm-flailing, and middle-finger waving to invalidate the otherwise accurate perception of Dan as an affable, cognitively sound, and emotionally stable relational partner. As deeply devoted to Dan as I am, those moments can be disruptive enough to pose a challenge—momentary though it is—to my own sense of our relationship; they are more corrosive to his status with those who are less bound to him by blood ties, lifelong history, and love. Because the frequency of those episodes to some degree reflects Dan's level of stress and aggravation, I had hoped he would experience fewer of them at Harbor than at Trinity Village, and he likely did, overall. But because life is inevitably stressful and aggravating at times (and life as a relatively young resident in a nursing home can be especially so), and because his neurological wiring reduces his ability to moderate his responses to stress and aggravation, Dan continued to struggle with his IED storms. Consequently, so did those around him.

Early on, I made a point of stressing to staff that Dan's explosive episodes are a common, if not universal, result of TBI that stems from organic disturbances beyond his control. I emphasized that his outbursts aren't something that he wills, but rather events he undergoes because of damaged circuitry in his brain. Explaining that they are the effects of neural impairment—tempests that blow through him, not tantrums he throws in a bid to get his own way—is one of the duties I viewed as indispensable to Dan's acceptance into his new community. I didn't hide the fact that, although I myself fully understand that in these moments he's in the grips of something he can't control, sometimes I'm unable to respond with the measured equilibrium rationally called for, and I lose my own composure. Obviously, I don't expect others to be unmoved by his rage attacks, which can feel unjust and deeply personal in the moment. Enduring those moments is hard, but the understanding that he is not in control of them does—or, at least in a perfect world, should—decrease whatever resentment might linger in their aftermath. There is no real "cure" for IED; the best we can hope for is to reduce the frequency of episodes by trying to avoid as much as possible the typical two-punch trigger: frustration at his lack of agency or control, combined with the sense of being diminished in some way by those he must depend upon for what he can't do for himself. And what can't be either fixed or avoided, by him or anyone else, must be borne with all the possible grace we can muster. But while understanding helps, it's not a panacea.

A key role I performed for Dan over those first few months was that of storyteller. When most of us are in the process of fostering new relationships, we share aspects of our lives that help others identify with us, developing the cognitive and emotional ties that lead to affiliation and mutual belongingness. Because of Dan's difficulty in communicating complex information, I made a point of sharing his life history with most of the personnel who came into contact with him, whatever their role. I outlined his oral paralysis, aphasia, IED, and anosognosia, all of which in the past had been consistently misinterpreted as signs of mental incompetence. I emphasized instead his acute awareness and sensitivity, his intelligence, his ability to understand everything that was said to him, and his capacity to respond and reciprocate through manual spelling and the laminated manual alphabet sheet. I elevator-speeched everyone who would listen about his accident, his persistent love of horses, and his subjection to chemical restraint at Trinity Village. I wanted the people charged with his care to understand his capabilities as well as his impairments and, especially, to *feel* for him. I wanted them not only to claim Dan as a responsibility but also to connect with him as an individual who still experienced the full range of human emotions—not just explosive rage. It was important to ensure, as effectively as I could, that Dan wouldn't just be *taken care of*, but would be *cared about*. I hoped to weave as much belongingness as possible into his life.

I counted on the power of narrative—the deep human reliance on story to make meaning of our experiences—to accomplish that goal. Human beings love stories, and without exception listeners responded to Dan's history with curiosity and empathy. Sometimes the stories were short, focusing on whatever past episodes from his life helped to illuminate his feelings or behavior or perspective in the present moment. At other times the accounts were more comprehensive, intended to give an overview of what Dan's life had been like both before and since his accident. In all cases, these chronicles were unscripted—spontaneously generated to adapt to the given moment—but, to various degrees both consciously and subconsciously, I aimed at good storytelling. The events of Dan's life provided an organically dramatic frame, with abundant material to choose from that conveyed his early dreams, his loves, his losses, his hard-won accomplishments, and his multifaceted character. The stories arose easily, emerging from our mutual connection and my desire to appropriately humanize him for others through his own experiences. And even though I did have a specific goal—to advance his acceptance—there was nothing manipulative or deceptive in the telling. I spoke sincerely, pulling threads from a complex of love, grief, anger, relief, and hope that had been shaped and reshaped over decades.

Soon after I began telling these stories, it occurred to me that, even though Dan was present for nearly every recounting, I might have been trespassing on his privacy by sharing his life history, especially by including so much detail. When I had the thought, after the first week or so, I asked him if he'd rather I stop, or at least include only more general information. He emphatically shook his head "NO." Did he think others having more background about him was making a difference? His nod was just as emphatic: "YES."

Most of us take for granted our ability to share our histories with others as a form of generating empathy and bonding. Dan hadn't been able to perform that essential task for forty years. And I'm sure he was right. Those around him having a good sense of who he is, because they know his story, makes a difference.

★ ★ ★

Early in Dan's transition from Trinity Village to Harbor, the details flew thick and fast. Three days after his arrival, Harbor held his first "care plan conference," a gathering of staff from various departments to discuss Dan's needs and to develop strategies for meeting them. The resident and family members are invited to attend, and Dan and I eagerly accepted the invitation. For this first meeting, Harbor staff included the chief administrator herself (Shiloh), the head physical therapist, the speech therapist, the dietician, and the facility's chaplain. I emailed Shiloh that night, noting the almost disorienting shift between Dan's life at Trinity Village and his initial experiences at Harbor, which the meeting seemed to encapsulate:

> [S]itting in that meeting today, with Dan surrounded by people who genuinely care about his well-being, who are both able and willing to help him, was an almost surreal experience. Given where we've been, it's almost as though we've landed on another planet. Everyone has been absolutely superb. We both—and also our older brother Dave, whom I've been briefing via email—are so very happy to have found Harbor Health. Thanks for all you do, and thanks for making the leap of faith that is making all of this possible for Dan.

By the end of his first week, Dan had a fresh haircut, a daily therapy schedule, and an appointment for a dental cleaning and checkup for the first time in a decade. He was receiving daily shaves and biweekly showers (the frequency he himself had chosen). His food preferences and interests had been recorded. Hates: fish, oatmeal, mashed potatoes, and spaghetti (difficult for him to chew and swallow). Loves: salads, cheeseburgers, pizza, burritos, fried clams, horses, and country music. For this interview, the social services person used the same form that the CNA at Trinity Village had dutifully charted with us in December, twelve years after he moved in and two months before he'd be moving out. Dan was getting out of bed every day, watching TV from a wheelchair, regaining strength and vitality, and pleasantly interacting with those who cared for him. It was a drastically different life from the one he'd left behind, immobilized in bed and staring at the ceiling.

All of these changes were positive, but the pervasiveness and degree of change were dramatic and therefore at times overwhelming. Dan was glad to be getting out of bed and showering, and yet, given the degree of frailty and enervation that had developed over months and even years of malnutrition and inactivity, those modest undertakings were painful. He asked me to relay to Harbor staff that, while he wasn't complaining or accusing them of carelessness or roughness, he was hoping they could minimize his discomfort if they were aware of it. Also, he found sitting up for extended periods both painful and exhausting, so he requested that he be moved into his chair for no more than hour-long intervals several times a day until he became accustomed to this new level of activity. Harbor was warmly responsive to our requests and demonstrated that, as Shiloh had promised, residents' choices—not staff convenience—shaped the rules and procedures that structured and so sculpted their daily lives.

Although I was well aware that IED is neither "curable" nor simply a function of external conditions, I was nevertheless dispirited by his first outburst, which gusted through him on his eighth day at Harbor. Due to a staffing issue, when a worker called in sick, breakfast was delayed. Dan assumed he'd been forgotten and erupted into a full-blown rage, sweeping everything off his bed table and spilling milk all over his bed. I detailed in my journal the discussion we shared later that afternoon:

> I talked to him for quite awhile, assuring him that he wouldn't be forgotten, pointing out that the staff is caring for many other people too and sometimes may take longer than he'd like to get to him. I reminded him that not only is it good to treat people well because it's the right thing to do, but it also serves us better because we catch more flies with honey than vinegar. It's simply human not to respond well when people yell at us and throw stuff—that the most likely outcome of that behavior is an attitude something like "Let him sit in that milk, then." Dan listened intently and agreed with me. I know he can't stop his reactions when he reaches those flashpoints, but I'm hoping that helping him view the situation differently—reminding him that people *do* care, that they *are* trying, that they *don't* view him as undeserving of attention or negligible because of his disabilities, and that *everyone* makes mistakes—can help him to avoid reaching those flashpoints in the first place.

I would discover later, in the course of researching this book, that encouraging Dan to think differently about the situations that generate his rages follows a foundational concept in cognitive behavioral therapy (CBT). A pragmatic approach to behavioral change, engaging in this kind of therapeutic program reportedly helps at least some TBI survivors manage their IED.

A couple of weeks later, someone in the kitchen forgot to add the evening's entrée, a Philly steak sandwich, to Dan's dinner tray. He was still hungry when I visited that evening, so I bought him a can of cashews to add to a stash of meal bars and cookies that Marjorie had assembled for him. We discussed the incident while he ate cashews. I recorded our talk in my journal that night:

> Dan believes he's being slighted because he's disabled and people don't think he's aware enough to matter—maybe they even want to be mean to him because of his disabilities. He feels he's treated as though he's like a "BABY," not "SMART." I assured him that no one is intentionally causing him problems—that things such as forgetting the entrée are nothing more nefarious than a mistake, and that the solution is to calmly remind people of what they've forgotten or to point out the mistake and give them an opportunity to correct it. He doesn't agree that these oversights are accidental. I was reminded of an experience we had back at Taylor Heights, where Mom, Dave, Dan, and I went to a Mexican restaurant for lunch, and Dan said (after the meal) that the ground beef in his meal tasted strange—and that he was given spoiled food because of his "HANDICAP." So he's still operating on the belief that people intentionally abuse him because of his disabilities. I don't know if that has ever happened to him, but if it has, surely it's been the exception rather than the rule, and I'd like to help him rethink and reframe this assumption.

The way he had been treated at Trinity Village constituted a sort of passive abuse; his chemical restraint testified to that. But active denigration or intentional mistreatment? Surely not! But I would later learn that indeed there are people who have directly, openly disparaged Dan because of his impairments—bullies who have belittled and mocked him simply because he could neither stop them nor defend himself. Why vulnerability arouses contempt in some people is beyond me. Why they not only entertain such disdain but also feel free to unleash it—why they are not constrained by a sense of decency, if empathy is too much to expect—is a further mystery. Abstractly, I have known for years that such people exist. But that someone would want—much less dare—to demean Dan, who so clearly has faced more than his share of misfortune, would prove as eye-opening to me as it was disturbing. It would drive home the lesson that Dan's occasional sense of victimization, which I had relegated to the category of "unjustified" by default, was perhaps grounded in experience. I can't know all that has happened to him over the past forty-plus years. And with his aphasia, coupled with a degree of apparently permanent memory loss as a result of chemical restraint, there is—and will remain—much that he can't tell me.

★ ★ ★

In early March, little more than two weeks after moving to Harbor, Dan told me that he was "LONELY," that some of the staff didn't speak to him at all when they came into his room, while others spoke to him as though he were a "BABY." People's perceptions of him as cognitively and emotionally incompetent, and the sense of isolation he experiences as a result, have been a chronic problem for Dan ever since his accident. No matter how much I explain that he is able both to understand whatever is said to him and to respond appropriately through manual spelling or his letter board, the tone of his interactions seems to be set by default by his inability to speak, coupled with the severity of his physical (e.g., visible) impairments. This pattern of interaction is dismaying but not surprising; although there is no necessary correlation among linguistic expression, physical soundness, and cognitive competence, we tend to assess others as though there were. Ever since his accident, Dan has been excluded from the social category of "normal," even though he more accurately belongs to a more complex classification: someone who is normal in some ways and atypical in others—a classification to which we all belong, to greater or lesser degrees.

I had noticed, and I affirmed in my conversation with Dan, that when others come into his room for whatever reason, when I'm present, they often speak *to* me and *of* him. He nodded vigorously. "I know that's a problem," I said. "People just don't know *how* to interact with you. It's not that they don't think you're worth talking to—although I suspect that may have been an issue for a few people you've dealt with." He nodded gravely. "But I would bet that, with most people, they just don't know how to communicate with you, and that makes them uncomfortable." He shrugged and lifted his palm—in effect, *I don't know what I can do to change that.* "I know it's hard," I said. "I know it wears on you. But let's give people time to learn. I'll keep trying to help people understand," I promised. "In the meantime, you just keep on being you. You're awesome, Dan. And, maybe not everybody, but at least some of these folks are going to realize that."

He shrugged again, but this time the shrug was accompanied by a warm smile and glittering eyes.

★ ★ ★

Dave's first visit to Harbor from his new home in Maryland coincided with Dan's fifty-eighth birthday. Dan was delighted to see his brother, and the three of us went to lunch in downtown Muncie. It was the first time Dan had wanted to participate in an excursion for about a year.

Although it was mid-March, fat snowflakes fell from a steely gray Indiana sky. Historically, Dan has been opposed to wearing long-sleeved shirts, jackets, or coats, so he was wearing the warmest piece of clothing he had: a fleece vest. But he was no longer in Southern California or Georgia. Gooseflesh pebbled his arms, his teeth chattered, and his cheeks were rouged by the cold air. "INDIANA COLD! SNOW!" he spelled, his shivering adding the exclamation points. But chilled though he certainly was—and as glad as he was when we finally pushed him through the doors into the warmth of the brew pub—even as we rushed him through the parking lot, with the soft flakes melting on his head, face, and arms, his bright laughter pealed across the asphalt.

★ ★ ★

Dan's second care conference a few days later was a series of glowing reports both from Harbor personnel and us; everyone was pleased by Dan's new situation. There was only one real problem that needed addressing, but it was a serious one that had caused difficulties at Trinity Village and that was arising again in his new home: Dan was having roommate troubles. The cause was the same too: temperature wars. Lest the ambient room temperature seemed like a small thing to clash over, I noted in the care conference (and everyone agreed) that any of us would be distressed if we had no control over the temperature within our own homes.

Until recently, by all reports Dan's new roommate, Albert, had been a soft-spoken, polite, easy-going octogenarian. However, he had recently begun developing dementia and was undergoing personality changes. My first encounter with him in February had been pleasant, as he murmured to me that he and Dan would get along just fine because, as he boasted with a subdued smile, he could "get along with anyone." Before the first week was over, though, conflict was brewing.

Dan, like many TBI survivors, is particularly sensitive to cold temperatures, and left to his own devices, he prefers his surroundings at a warm and toasty 76°. Albert, however, wanted the temperature a good ten degrees cooler. As I learned at the care plan conference, Harbor had negotiated a compromise between Dan and Albert: the thermostat would remain set at 70°.

Initially, the agreement seemed to work. Dan found 70° a tad chilly but bearable if he bundled up, and he endured the cooler temperature with stoic good grace. Albert, though, huddling under a pile of blankets on his side of the room, took to muttering obscenities while grousing about the heat, which Dan found by turns amusing and irritating.

Dan was incensed, however, when Albert began flouting their pact by breezing past Dan to lower the thermostat. Since Dan couldn't propel himself in his wheelchair to restore the setting to 70°, his only recourse was to summon a nurse or CNA with his call button, so that they could intervene on his behalf. This unpleasantness continued for a week or two. The nurses and CNAs were increasingly exasperated, since they had enough to do without having to repeatedly address the situation, and Dan was ever more frustrated and furious. By transgressing their agreement, Albert was violating Dan's sense of fair play and, perhaps even more inflammatory, underscoring his helplessness. It was deeply humiliating for Dan not to be able to prevent a cognitively failing octogenarian from exerting his will by trampling on Dan's.

Tensions further escalated after Albert realized he could circumvent staff intervention by resetting Dan's call light before anyone had a chance to see it. When Dan pressed the button to summon help, Albert would turn the call light off by disconnecting the plug and reconnecting it, so that no one was the wiser. Because the outlet was behind a curtain on Albert's side of the room, his subterfuge initially went undetected. For days, Dan was phoning me to angrily report that his call light was going unheeded. Since feeling helpless and disregarded was one of the predictable triggers for his IED, tensions were mounting on every side. In response to Dan's complaints, I was calling the nurse's desk inquiring about the inordinate length of time he was waiting for a response to his call light. Repeatedly I was told that his light wasn't on—and yes, it was working, so perhaps he wasn't using the button correctly? A week or so into this spiraling dynamic, a CNA caught Albert in the act of unplugging Dan's light, and the mystery was solved.

Albert was told that such stunts could endanger Dan's health and safety and simply wouldn't be tolerated. But he was unwilling or unable to restrain himself, and a day or two later, I walked into Dan's room to a flurry of activity as Albert's belongings were being packed into boxes. He was moved to another room in another section of the building, and we never saw him again.

For several months, we waited to see who would take Albert's place, hoping that Dan's new roommate would cooperate in making the environment livable for both of them. That summer, however, Harbor reclassified all of the rooms on Dan's hall as single occupancy. As a result, Dan continued to enjoy the privacy, the expanded space, and the warmth of having the room all to himself.

★ ★ ★

By all accounts, dental anxiety is a real condition. For Dan, though, his first trip to the dentist in over a decade was cause for celebration.

Marjorie made the appointment for him with her own dentist and arranged transportation.

It was a fine but chilly spring morning in April, two months after Dan's arrival at Harbor. Our mood was festive. I stood back as Dan in his wheelchair was lifted, strapped, and buckled into the van, a stress-free, streamlined process which took only minutes. I admired and appreciated the driver's expertise as he deftly operated the lift and adjusted the myriad hooks and belts while chattering amiably about the weather and his love for his job. Some fifteen minutes later, I was pushing Dan's wheelchair through the double glass doors of the dental complex.

I handed a large manila envelope containing Dan's Medicare information to the desk attendant, who passed me a clipboard holding new patient forms. Dan and I moved off to the side of the large carpeted lobby to fill out the paperwork together. When I returned the forms to the desk, the attendant told me that she hadn't been able to verify Dan's Medicare coverage; was I sure he had been cleared for this dental visit? No, I said, I don't know anything about the paperwork or the financial arrangements, but if there were any problems, the office could bill me— and I gave her my name and address. I was fairly certain that the charges would be covered by Medicare, but nothing was going to stop Dan from getting his teeth cleaned and examined that morning. If billing issues arose, I'd sort them out later. (For the record, there were no issues, and I was never charged.)

Dan and I didn't wait long before Melissa, the dental technician, beckoned us into a luminescent labyrinthine hallway. We followed her into a treatment cubby gleaming with chrome. "I see in your chart, Dan, that you haven't seen a dentist in about ten years, is that right?" she asked. Dan nodded in response.

I was glad that she addressed her question to Dan and not to me, but I felt it was important to explain that his lapse in dental care was not because he was disinterested but because it had been denied him. In fact, I noted, I learned on the night of Dan's arrival in Muncie that Trinity Village staff hadn't given him the opportunity to brush his teeth for eight months or so before he left their facility. Setting him up so that he could brush his teeth twice a day was one of Dan's first requests at Harbor. "I'd be willing to bet big money," I told Melissa, "that, of all your patients, Dan's one of the happiest ever to be here." Dan grinned and nodded.

Melissa kept up a friendly patter as she prepped her instruments and adjusted equipment to accommodate Dan's wheelchair. The angle of the wheelchair's back was adjustable, so he didn't need to transfer into the dental chair; I lowered the back so that it was nearly parallel to the floor, and Melissa swung the overhead lamp to illuminate Dan's mouth, which he opened wide. She inspected his teeth and poked his gums before getting down to the business of scraping, whirring, and buffing. A few minutes after she finished, the dentist arrived to assess the state of Dan's teeth. When he read in the chart that Dan hadn't received dental care in more than ten years, he was astonished that there wasn't a mouthful of problems to address. I offered the fact that Dan seldom ate sweets, and the dentist acknowledged that the good decisions Dan made about his diet were likely responsible for his remarkably healthy teeth. Dan nodded, beaming. The dentist recommended that Dan return in six weeks for a second cleaning, in light of the long interval his mouth had gone without attention, and again praised him for the healthy dietary choices that had helped maintain his dental health. Dan fairly glowed under the praise.

As we waited for the transport van that would return us to Harbor, during a pause in our conversation, Dan reached for my hand and squeezed it, meeting my eye with a glittering smile. Getting my teeth cleaned is something I do every six months or so. It's a routine part of my life, predictable and a bit tedious, grudgingly accepted as a necessary unpleasantness. Not so for Dan. This trip to the dentist was a red-letter day for him. He was receiving the care he had longed for but that he'd been unable to obtain. Going to the dentist signaled a deeper shift in his life: he was working his way back into the ordinary activities of normal life and re-entering a complex of customary community relationships that he had lost, one by one, over time. Since earliest childhood, I had taken for granted this interlaced network and the quotidian activities that build and sustain it, viewing them as simply an inherent and therefore predictable part of existence. For Dan, this re-entry was a renewal. He was rejoining the ranks for whom affirmed dignity was a baseline expectation. My hope was that I could help him assume a place within the societal complex that made a trip to the dentist, and the affirmation by erstwhile strangers of his fundamental worth as a fellow human being, wholly unremarkable.

★ ★ ★

In mid-May, Harbor held a special "Farm Animal Day." Several families from the surrounding countryside transported some of their animals—a goat, a sheep, a calf, a pair of chickens, and two horses—to Harbor's parking lot, where residents gathered to greet and pet them. I asked Dan if he was interested in visiting with the animals, and he nodded but added a shrug to signal nonchalance; the message was, Sure, I'll go, but it would be silly to get excited over a few barnyard chickens. When Dan saw the horses, though, all insouciant posturing disappeared. His delight in the presence of the two horses, TC and Cimarron, was unfiltered; he lit up with it. He established an immediate bond with Cim. Dan stroked the animal's muzzle with the easy assurance of an inveterate horseman, and Cim responded by nuzzling his hand and snuffling his hair, gladdening everyone in the vicinity, but especially Dan. Back in the presence of a horse—the sensory extravagance of Cim's distinctively equine aroma, his coarse but glossy coat, sweet grain breath and inquisitive, quivering muzzle, friendly brown eyes, and insistent nose-nudges requesting more rubs—for those brief moments, Dan forgot everything else: all of his sadnesses and hardships, his rejections and dejections. It all just melted like snow in the soft May evening, leaving nothing but Dan's pure, clean love of HORSE.

★ ★ ★

In June, Dyke and I bought a condo in Muncie. For nearly two years, we had been considering relocating there from Fishers, which is why I sought a facility for Dan in Muncie, rather than in our Indianapolis bedroom community some forty-five miles away. Dyke's job was nearer to Muncie than to Fishers, and mine was the same distance from either town, so our overall time commuting for work would be reduced. Besides, we were driving to Muncie once or twice on most weekends already. I had been attending church there for several years, and for much of that time, I actively volunteered on the state re-election campaigns for a fellow church member and friend. Unrelated political work had led to Dyke's and my membership in the Muncie chapter of the League of Women Voters. As a result, most of our acquaintances and nearly all of our non-workplace friends lived in Muncie. While we loved our house in Fishers, it was located in the reddest county in the overwhelmingly red state of Indiana, and we didn't fit in politically with the vast majority of our neighbors. I hoped that a move to purple Muncie, where we were already spending much of our extracurricular time, would help us to feel a more integral part of the community and so to find the greater sense of belonging I longed for.

For well over a year, Dyke and I had been dabbling in house-hunting, enjoying it as a comfortable hobby. We ritualized our Sunday afternoons after church with a lunch buffet at a local Indian restaurant followed by leisurely drives through various neighborhoods, punctuated by explorations of an occasional open house that seemed promising. We dreamed and discussed, neither of us in any hurry to conclude a process that we were finding so pleasant.

But once Dan arrived in Muncie, when I was commuting to and from Harbor after each workday as well as on Saturdays and Sundays, I experienced a skyrocketing sense of urgency to move. Dyke and I doubled down, focusing on neighborhoods within a fifteen-minute drive from Harbor. Within four months of Dan's arrival, we had closed on a condo twelve minutes from his new home, shifting our base of operations.

Dyke's role in helping to upgrade Dan's lot with relocation to Harbor, and his engagement in the subsequent push to improve Dan's life, can't be overstated. This process has been, and continues to be, time intensive and emotionally absorbing, and Dyke's and my life together has changed in ways both large and small. Dyke has assisted me in scaling each wall, in salving each bruise. Most dramatically, though, his willingness to abort our search for the "right" house—to scale down from our perfect house in Fishers to a smaller, older condo in Muncie because it brought us nearer to Dan's residence—reveals the depth of his commitment to both Dan and me. Dyke has been a willing partner in ensuring not only that his brother-in-law is safe but that he feels prioritized and well supported. He's unmistakably increased the measure of Dan's belongingness. And, to a degree impossible to express, mine too.

★ ★ ★

Dan continued to settle in nicely. That spring, he asked for a bird feeder. I set a tiered pole outside his window and adorned it with a cottage-style feeder and a small hanging cedar birdbath. In good weather, he accompanied me outside into the courtyard twice a week to refill the feeder and bath, carrying the bag of seed and a plastic gallon jug of water on his lap. After the first couple of months, he upgraded to the deluxe seed mix, a richer blend that cost more but that brought more birds to his window and reduced how often the feeder needed refilling (which he kept a close eye on). Finches and sparrows swooped and darted, shoving each other out of the way as they hopped along the rim of the feeder, exuberantly spraying seed as they dipped their beaks into the feeder slots. Dan reveled in the show, and also in the knowledge that he was supporting the birds, especially those who wintered over despite Indiana's snow and ice. Providing them all, year-round, with life-sustaining food and water allowed him to contribute materially to the world—more specifically, to the bright-eyed little creatures whose visits bestowed so much pleasure. Helping them was no small thing to either of us, and it gratified us both.

★ ★ ★

By the time fall semester began in late August at the community college where I taught full-time, Dan was comfortable with cutting back the frequency of our visits from daily to biweekly. We soon established an agreeable groove. On Sundays, it became Dyke's and my custom to bring Dan a lunch of his choosing, usually a cheeseburger, although he occasionally asked to shake up the routine by substituting a burrito or a pepperoni pizza. Dyke and I watched AMC or the NFL channel with him while he ate. Aligning with my teaching schedule, Wednesdays were set aside for less structured visits, which we used to address occasional questions or issues as they arose. When the weather was fine, we'd go into the courtyard to feed the birds, lingering to get some sun and gaze at the lone hawk who frequently spiraled or hung suspended in the blue sky above Harbor's roofline. On both visiting days, I delivered incidental supplies and performed little chores as needed. I now lived nearby if Dan needed unscheduled help, but he seldom did. I was increasingly less often called upon to run interference—either by Dan for help with Harbor staff or by Harbor staff for help with Dan—and I could typically address any issues that came up with a phone call or two. I phoned Dan at least twice a day—every morning when I woke up and every night just before he went to sleep. These phone calls mostly served to touch base, reassuring me that Dan was fine, and reassuring Dan that, although I was less often physically present, I was no less engaged, and he remained a top priority.

Dan was considerably more comfortable than he had been at Trinity Village, and the adjustments and re-adjustments remained ongoing. When his room was declared single occupancy, and therefore his own space, we further personalized it by hanging more pictures and photographs. He got a small refrigerator for storing leftovers and condiments, which enabled him to exercise his eating and drinking preferences—selection, timing, and frequency—in ways that had never occurred to me to consider, reminding me yet again of how much I take for granted in my own life. And that fall, he bought a warm coat, which I took to a tailor for a sleeve alteration to accommodate the braces on his right arm. The Indiana "COLD" no longer loomed quite so uncomfortably.

Not everything worked out flawlessly. Dave hauled Dan's motorized wheelchair up from Georgia, and we had it reconditioned for Dan's use at Harbor. But during the therapy department's evaluation to certify his ability to safely operate the chair, Dan erupted with an IED storm. Consequently, and especially given his record at Trinity Village, he was denied approval to use it, a verdict that initially incensed him. He insisted that, since the chair belonged to him, no one else had a right to prevent him from using it whenever and wherever he wanted. After some discussion, he accepted, if not the justness of the decision, Harbor's right to make it. At that point, he requested that he be scheduled for re-evaluation after going six months without an outburst. The head therapist agreed. Unfortunately (but predictably), he was unable to remain episode-free for six weeks. As a result, the chair sat in a corner of his room more than three years later. At some point none of us noticed, the ($500) battery disappeared.

Still, within six months of his arrival at Harbor, Dan's life had vastly improved. He was receiving rounds of physical and occupational therapy, which were helping him recover some of the strength and functionality he had lost as a result of chemical restraint and eight months in bed. He had gained thirty pounds; not only did he no longer need to drink the supplemental shakes he so despised, but he was watching his diet so that he wouldn't gain more weight. He felt better; he looked better; he *was* better.

Still, Dan's new story had just begun.

8 Finding Agape

Until July of 2018, I had never heard of OBRA, which is an acronym for the Omnibus Budget Reconciliation Act, a federal bill signed into law in 1987. Also known as the Nursing Home Reform Act, OBRA aims to foster conditions that enable nursing home residents to "attain and maintain [their] highest practicable physical, mental, and psychosocial well-being."[1] Its provisions established national minimum standards that long-term care facilities are required to meet, along with a roster of rights guaranteed to residents in their care. Focusing not only on facility practices that safeguard health and safety, the act mandates that "[a] nursing facility must care for its residents in such a manner and in such an environment as will promote maintenance or enhancement of the quality of life of each resident."[2] In other words, OBRA stresses quality of life as well as quality of care.

Along with a number of important reforms to long-term care facility practices (including the prohibition of chemical restraint when used for "purposes of discipline or convenience and not required to treat the resident's medical symptoms"[3]), OBRA's emphasis on the psychosocial well-being and life enrichment of residents entitled Dan to receive specialized services, namely support in the form of personal assistance so that he could regularly participate in activities beyond Harbor Health's walls, like trips to restaurants or to movie theaters.

I found out about OBRA through a phone call, completely unexpected, that I received from a local OBRA service coordinator. Her job, Carrie told me, was to determine the eligibility of potential clients and to arrange the provision of services for those who qualified and wanted to take part in the program. After briefly explaining to me what that meant, Carrie asked me if I thought Dan might be interested.

I could hardly speak. I had never dreamed, much less heard, of any such program, and the prospect of connecting Dan to services that would enable him to engage regularly in the kinds of experiences most of us take

DOI: 10.4324/9781003340294-8

for granted was electrifying. The world suddenly expanded, as decades-long barriers seemed poised to tumble like dominoes, steamrolled by promise. From the moment Dan regained consciousness after his accident, he wanted nothing more than to feel (and be regarded as) normal again. As Carrie described it (although not in these terms), OBRA services would boost him closer to the experience of "normal" than he'd been able to reach in a long time. Of course I would have to check with Dan before committing him to anything, but I told Carrie that I couldn't imagine a scenario in which he would decline an opportunity like this.

Something in the conversation stuck in my mind, though, worrying me at the edges of thought. It took me a few moments to identify it. The term *developmental disabilities*, to me, suggested congenital impairment, like Down's syndrome or autism. If that were the case, I told Carrie, Dan wouldn't qualify for the program because his impairments had been acquired long after childhood. Carrie explained to me that a variety of conditions are considered "developmental" if they arise before adulthood, and brain injury is one of them. Because Dan's TBI occurred when he was still a teenager, he was indeed eligible for OBRA services. I was thrilled and could hardly wait to tell Dan.

A week later, Dan and I gathered around a table in a conference room at Harbor with Carrie, one of Harbor's social services representatives, and two administrators from an agency called Indiana Friends, which would be contracted to provide the transportation and personal assistance that would facilitate Dan's excursions into the community.

Within the first few minutes of the meeting, I offered a brief but comprehensive narrative of Dan's history, including a thumbnail survey of his pre-accident life, the accident itself, and the various circumstances he'd lived in since. I emphasized Dan's intelligence and his alertness, but I also offered a condensed explanation of the IED and anosognosia that have caused him such difficulty since his accident. I pointed out that others' responses to those impairments—organic problems that he is unable, not unwilling, to control—had driven the kinds of painful and life-threatening marginalization Dan had experienced, emblematized by Trinity Village's chemical restraint. I noted how much his life had improved in the five months he'd lived at Harbor, and how grateful both he and I were for the difference. I added that we were excited by the prospect of OBRA services and that we appreciated how greatly expeditions into the Muncie community would weave more interest and enjoyment into the life he was rebuilding.

After learning what to expect from the program, Dan signed the necessary paperwork, which Carrie promised to submit that afternoon. She didn't anticipate any problems and expected that the funding would be secured within a few weeks. Then the expeditions would begin. It was almost too good to believe. The glow that diffused the conference room, these near strangers enveloping Dan in a honeyed haze of warm regard, felt nothing short of miraculous.

★ ★ ★

Dan's outings with Indiana Friends began in mid-August of 2018, six months after his arrival at Harbor in February. Dan and I had been tasked with putting together a list of activities he would enjoy doing, and we repeatedly tried to compose one, but our list remained woefully short. Other than going to lunch and the movies, he either lacked interest or was physically unable to participate in the kinds of pursuits we could think of. He wasn't interested in trips to shopping malls, museums, or parks. Being passively pushed through aisles or along walkways would provide a change of scenery, but it also would undermine the sense of autonomy and relative normalcy he was constantly striving for. We brainstormed frequently, but community offerings that matched Dan's interests and abilities were sparse.

The first Indiana Friends staff person assigned to accompany Dan on outings was an energetic woman in her sixties. I met her in Dan's room just before their first expedition, a scheduled lunch outing. She was both steely and cheery, with a "can-do" spirit and a nonstop patter that I found a bit overwhelming. She told Dan and me that the people in her charge had been given up on by everyone else, but, under her care and with her encouragement, even these unfortunates could "do anything," and she had the success stories to prove it. One dispirited little girl with cerebral palsy, she recounted, had been bereft of hope because everyone else in her life told her that she was weak and helpless, but this woman had changed that little girl's life. Under her tutelage, that fearful little girl realized that she could accomplish anything she wanted to. And so she conquered her fears, and did.

I was uneasy about this story on several fronts. First, Dan had never been viewed by his family as (or told by us that he was) incapable of pursuing his goals, except as they concerned using a wheelchair instead of buddy-walking, which actually increased rather than diminished his level of independence, and abandoning his tenacious hope of driving again, which may have prevented injuries or death (including, but not necessarily only, his). Aside from that, we encouraged his efforts to reach the goals he set. I had to admit, though, that we may not have always proactively sought ways to help him broaden those boundaries, some of which were perhaps more permeable than we had understood them to be.

Also, it struck me as dangerous to tell a TBI survivor with anosognosia that there was nothing he couldn't do, that he was limited only by other people who refused to see his potential. I certainly didn't want to undermine whatever efforts Dan undertook to improve himself—and in fact I wanted to encourage him to set goals and reach them, and to arrange external conditions that would optimize his success and happiness. But I also didn't want him to overreach sensible safeguards that reduced his risk of further injury or to harbor truly unrealistic expectations that could only end in disappointment, frustration, or anger. It was—and remains—important for those who work with Dan to recognize his possibilities, but it's equally important that he respect efforts to ensure his safety. We all have limitations. And limitations are real and organic, not just imagined by others because of their lack of faith in us.

In short, I didn't want anyone encouraging him to endanger his own well-being or to set him up for failure. And I didn't want those around Dan blamed if he was unable to reach every goal he set for himself. Because of the neurological disconnection between his awareness of his impairments and his grasp of the limitations they impose, Dan continually dances on the fine line dividing possibility from impossibility. This woman's insistence that he could do anything he put his mind to suggested that he would achieve even his most impracticable goals, except to the degree that others stood in his way. If Dan took this exhortation to heart, everyone who tried to help him accommodate his intransigent neurological impairments—to adapt to them, or to work around rather than through them—would be placed in the category of hindrance. And that would certainly include me.

As it turned out, I didn't have to worry about his new assistant's influence for long. Dan didn't care much for her overbearing interactive style or for most of the outings she took him on. Her idea of lunch, for example, consisted of a milkshake from the drive-through at Dairy Queen, which he drank in his wheelchair, belted and strapped into the back of an agency van, as she drove around the city streets for a couple of hours. After several bored and hungry afternoons, he asked if he could change assistants.

Still, Dan's brief stint with his first personal assistant had an unexpected consequence that, as it turned out, would prove life-changing. In preparation for working with Dan, she had been briefed about his history, including his history with horses and his unflagging love for them. She knew a family on the outskirts of Muncie who owned a couple of horses, and she arranged to drop by their barn with Dan. On this visit, as on Harbor's Farm Animal Day, he was practically reborn in their company, both soothed and invigorated by their touch, their smell, their very presence.

For the first months of OBRA outings, Carrie frequently contacted me to evaluate how well the program was meeting Dan's needs. After the first few weeks, I noted that he enjoyed the movies, didn't care much for the "lunches," but had absolutely delighted in the barn visit. Early in the fall, Carrie phoned me with an exhilarating prospect: she had scouted the region and discovered Agape Therapeutic Riding Center in Cicero, about an hour's drive from Muncie. Agape, she told me, was a nonprofit organization that offered horseback riding lessons as a means of cultivating strength, balance, and self-confidence for people with impairments (as well as for seniors and at-risk youth). Did that sound like a program that might interest Dan?

I was almost too thrilled to speak. I knew Dan would embrace this potential opportunity, and I was right. By December, we had arranged an appointment in the first week of January to evaluate his physical ability to participate in Agape's program. Dan was ecstatic, and so was I—despite a forewarning from the site's director, Amy, that not everyone who applied was capable of passing the assessment, which was aimed at ensuring participants' safety. From what I had told Amy of Dan's physical condition, she was skeptical that he could manage the demands of riding, but she was certainly hoping that he could. I appreciated her effort to remain (and to keep Dan and me) simultaneously optimistic and grounded in reality, which almost certainly, in her line of work (as well as in our experience), more than occasionally proved bitter.

★ ★ ★

Harbor held its Christmas party in early December. In most ways, it was like the event the year before. The halls and dining tables were cheerily decked. Personnel, residents, and family members were merry and bright, variously adorned with Santa hats, spangled sweaters, and even blinking lights affixed to their persons. The karaoke-singing saxophonist had returned to spin his DVDs and nod modestly to acknowledge his audience's applause. The salad, rolls, green beans, mashed potatoes, and pumpkin pie were again nothing special, but nevertheless something special.

Despite the similarities, though, this year's gathering was significantly different. This time we were with Dan, in his new home, in his new community. We were no longer prospective members of that community; we were an accepted part of it. We knew many of the staff members' names, some of their stories, and nearly all of their faces, and they knew ours. Pleasantries were more spontaneous and warmer, more personal. We were no longer strangers, wondering why, exactly, we'd been invited.

We were celebrating Christmas, of course, but this time we were also celebrating belongingness—all of ours together. Dan belonged, and so did we. The night shimmered.

★ ★ ★

Monday morning, January 7, 2019, began inauspiciously. We received a call from Indiana Friends reporting that the lift on their transport van wasn't working, so the agency had no way of getting Dan to Agape for his assessment. But the appointment was too important to him (and me) to be postponed. So with the help of a Harbor CNA, Dan transferred into my Prius, I folded down the back seats, and she and I crammed his wheelchair into the back compartment.

It was a fine winter day, the cloudless sky a soft powder blue. Dan and I zipped across a tawny landscape of beige-stubbled fields rimmed with brush and gray-boned trees. I cranked up the heater and iTunes, and we bobbed along to old country classics by Johnny Cash, Willie Nelson, and Waylon Jennings. We chalked up the miles as the hour flew by, and almost before we knew it, we pulled into Agape's gravel driveway, which curved around a corral where a band of horses stood munching their breakfast from buckets.

With some difficulty, Dan and I transferred him from the front seat to his wheelchair. I was guiding the wheelchair across the parking lot when Amy emerged from the building to greet us. When I told her who we were, she responded with an uncertain smile.

"You look a little surprised," I said.

"I am," she answered. "I guess there's been some kind of mix-up. Dan's assessment isn't until Thursday."

I'm sure my shoulders fell, but I took a breath, then shrugged. "Well, then, we'll be back Thursday," I said, and Dan and I headed back to the car. It was indeed a disappointment; we'd been looking forward to clearing the assessment hurdle—and to eliminating the uncertainty about how well Dan would do. But, as I told him, the timeline had been extended by only three days. We could view today's excursion as a leisurely jaunt through the countryside on a perfectly crystalline, crisp winter day.

So Dan and I clambered back into the Prius, where Willie and Waylon sang us back to Muncie. The sun poured down its white-gold light as the naked trees flew past, and we felt only slightly less buoyant than we had an hour earlier, when we'd been headed toward Agape and its prospective gift of horses.

★ ★ ★

Fortunately, Indiana Friends's van was fully operational by Thursday. Dan was in high spirits as his new attendant strapped him into the roomy rear area. I assumed a seat diagonally across from him, and we settled in for the ride. The trip was a bit bumpy, but the large windows streamed with sunlight and as we rattled along, I jabbered brightly, nearly shouting over the din and taking photos of Dan on my phone to send to Dave and Dyke.

This time, Amy and a cluster of volunteers were expecting us in the indoor vestibule leading to a covered arena. They fitted Dan with a helmet, which he reluctantly submitted to. However, that reluctance escalated into angry refusal when Amy and the volunteers prepared to lift him onto a dummy horse. Its painted eyes and artificial mane and tail infuriated him, too reminiscent of a child's rocking horse. He suddenly felt humiliated—definitely not what he signed up for. Hands shaking with anger, he spelled "NO BABY" and erupted into full-blown IED fury: hollering uncontrollably, red-faced, limbs stiffened, middle finger waving.

I tried to calm Dan down by assuring him that no one meant to insult him, noting that sitting on the mock horse was required for everyone who wanted to participate in Agape's program. But he was already in the throes of rage, unable to listen or care. "Okay, we'll leave then, Dan," I said. Both crushed and embarrassed, I assumed Amy and the volunteers would never agree to work with him after his explosion. "I'm sorry we wasted your time," I said. "We were really hoping this would work out."

But clearly this wasn't Amy's first rodeo. She smiled at me and waited for Dan's storm to subside. After a few moments, when his anger had ebbed, Dan lowered his head, tucking his face into his hand. "He's saying he's embarrassed and sorry," I said.

"No, we're sorry, Dan. We didn't mean to make you feel bad," she said. "This is just the first part of the assessment. Are you ready?" Dan nodded, and the volunteers lifted him from his wheelchair and onto the horse mockup.

"You passed," Amy said with a bright smile. "Ready to get up on a real horse?"

Dan nodded, returning her smile as he was helped back into his wheelchair. We entered the horse-mounting area of the arena, and I pushed him up a ramp to a wooden platform some four feet off the ground. A smaller platform, accessed by stairs, opposed it, leaving a space for the horse to stand between them. One of the volunteers slowly led a patient bay horse into the gap. When Dan was asked if he were ready to mount the horse, he signaled that he was.

Amy, with the help of several volunteers, lifted Dan carefully and lowered him gently onto the horse. I stood on the small platform, adjusting

Dan's leg on that side in an effort to seat him more squarely on the horse's back. His hips were too stiff to allow his knees to open widely enough to straddle the horse, and so his legs remained above the horse's spine, knees hovering over the animal's neck. Dan squinted in pain but, when asked if he wanted to discontinue the assessment, he shook his head. Amy wedged a Boppy pillow—a thick, u-shaped cushion—behind Dan's hips to help support him. The crew gingerly led the horse away from the mounting platform and into the riding arena, with Dan lying nearly supine upon the horse's back, his shoulders rising only slightly above the back ridge of the saddle. Two people on each side of the horse held Dan's hips and shoulders as the horse plodded a slow path around the arena a few times. The walkers continually struggled to keep Dan from sliding off the horse's back and tumbling to the ground, and I knew they were nervous by the way my own breath kept catching in my chest. I walked in front of, beside, and behind the group, documenting Dan's posture with a profusion of photos and snippets of video taken from all angles with my phone.

Not surprisingly, after fifteen minutes or so of evaluating Dan as he bobbed uncomfortably on the animal's back, Amy told Dan that Agape would not be able to offer him lessons until certain aspects of his physical condition improved. She pointed out that he had required five helpers to safely conduct him around the ring, but Agape had enough personnel to provide only two volunteers—three at most—on an ongoing basis. Dan would need to gain more flexibility in his hips and knees to straddle the horse more securely, and to strengthen his left arm so that he could hold on to the horn at the front of the saddle's pommel. Finally, he needed to strengthen his core muscles so that he could support and balance more of his own weight. After six months of working on these issues with Harbor's therapists, Amy said, he could return for another assessment if he wished.

Dan was disappointed but, offered the opportunity to try again, not daunted. The next day, I relayed Amy's concerns, along with the raft of photos and video clips I had taken, to Harbor's therapy department. The physical and occupational therapists pledged to devise a course of rehabilitation specifically aimed at enabling Dan to ride a horse. The plan was in place.

I didn't have to sell Dan on the hope that it would all work out. He was determined and began working tirelessly to re-enter the world of horses. With the assistance of Harbor's rehabilitation professionals, he knew beyond any doubt that he would—oh yes, he *would*—ride again.

★ ★ ★

A week later, while rummaging through boxes still unpacked since Dyke and I moved to Muncie the previous summer, I came across two photos. The first is black and white, showing Dan at fifteen years old, astride Dusty, the handsome palomino he'd bought with his earnings from Carbon Canyon Stables. He and Dusty had been photographed in the aftermath of winning a ribbon at a horse show. Dan, in a broad-brimmed Western hat, patterned Western shirt with pearl snaps, silver-spangled chaps, and gleaming boots, sits ramrod straight, solemn and proud, on Dusty's saddled back. The second photo, Dan's high school senior portrait, is in color, and it shows a young man in radiant health. His skin is clear and smooth, his cheeks and mouth flushed a deep rosy red, brown eyes bright with introspective intelligence and vitality. His expression is again solemn, but an irrepressible warmth plays at his lips and eyes. This photo was taken at Chelsea High School, a week before Dan's accident on Will Swift's ranch. Mom and Dad received the senior photos packet while the family was at the hospital in Tulsa, over a month before Dan regained consciousness.

I bought a pair of polished wood frames for the pictures. Neither photo was in pristine condition, but the flaws were barely noticeable once framed. I worked first on the one of Dan and Dusty. When I began to frame the other, I realized that some of what I thought was damage to the photo was actually a bit of dust and goo that had accumulated over the past four decades since the accident. As I carefully cleaned the photo with a moistened rag, Dan came into sharper focus, losing some of the blur that had obscured him. Sharpening the image was as simple as blotting and brushing off the dust, rather than just inserting the photo, as it was, into the frame. A little attention made a lot of difference.

The next day, I added the two photos to the montage of framed portraits, snapshots, and posters on the walls in Dan's room. Several Harbor staff members had brought him gifts which harmonized with the new additions: a large wall calendar, each month featuring sleek horses in seasonal natural settings; a poster of a racehorse that belonged to Adam, Harbor's director of nursing, the horse's well-shaped head filling the entire field; a thick steel horseshoe, which we nailed above the protective jockey helmet Mom and Dad had given Dan during his initial rehabilitation, now mounted on the wall over his TV. With each addition, Dan can be seen a bit more clearly. He's still proud and still, as ever, horse-crazy.

★ ★ ★

Dan and I had just finished reading Chapter Four of Lawrence Scanlan's *Wild About Horses*, a chapter called "The Gentle Art of the Horse Whisperer."[4] As Scanlan notes, "unmanageable" horses panic, bucking and biting in resistance to captivity. The traditional method of "breaking" a horse is a matter of demonstrating human domination over them by escalating their terror while proving to them the futility of trying to escape it. The primary lesson is that they are entirely dependent for safety on the goodwill of their captors, that they themselves are no longer able to obey their instincts, follow their inclinations, or control the circumstances that compose their destiny, and they have no hope of regaining their claim to freedom. It is the horse's spirit that breaks, as all hope for liberty and self-direction is shattered.

"Gentling" a horse, on the other hand, is a process of establishing trust and mutual respect between the horse and the "whisperer," who mindfully adopts the horse's point of view in order to understand their thoughts and emotions. The whisperer's aim is to *prevent* terror, to appropriately respond to what the horse is thinking and feeling in order to help them adjust to their new (admittedly unfair, desperately unwelcome) situation. Trust is essential, because the key is persuasion rather than force. Knowing when and how to interact with the horse, and when to leave them alone, giving them time to process their thoughts and feelings, is a skill born of empathy and a desire (not just a "willingness") to enter into their mental world, to intimately understand what they're going through. Horses can't talk, but they can and do communicate, whether those around them are sufficiently motivated to understand them or not. Ignoring, or worse still using against them, *what* they communicate—what they're thinking and feeling—isn't just counterproductive; it's inhumane.

I was struck by the correlation between the situation captive horses find themselves in—thrust into a world that seeks to "tame" them, to make them pliable; a world where others dominate, reordering their lives and ignoring or punishing protests that arise from pain, fear, or impotent anger; a world in which they are at the mercy of others who are focused solely on compliance, viewing the desire for liberty and self-governance as an obstacle to be obliterated, precluding the negotiated give-and-take that characterizes "gentling"—and Dan's position at Trinity Village. I'm sure that Trinity Village administrators and other personnel would bitterly bristle at the suggestion that their aim was to "break" or "tame" Dan, but however they would phrase it, their intent was inarguably to make him "manageable." In the end, when they couldn't force him to "behave" as they wished, they asserted their dominance. Rather than accommodating his needs for respect and a sense of his own agency—and the self-respect that relies to a substantial degree on fulfilling those needs—they immobilized him with drugs, subverting his will and abolishing his agency. They left Dan no doubt: he was fully in their hands and at their mercy.

As his experience at Harbor has demonstrated, a more effective (and, crucially, less brutal) strategy for encouraging Dan's concession to facility rules and routines is to respectfully enter into his mental space and interact with him accordingly. Except in cases where others might be endangered, Dan has regained the freedom to determine his own actions and activities, both large and small. And he has no more desire to endanger others than does any other responsible citizen. If a given behavior might put someone else's safety at risk, an explanation revealing the angle he hadn't considered is enough to sway him to alter his conduct, even if he doesn't agree that concern is warranted.

As I've noted before, Dan's outbursts often appear to be triggered by the obstruction of an intention, as a response to the frustration and anger he feels when his sense of agency is transgressed. He often experiences the actions of others that thwart him (even when those actions are justifiable) as a declaration of domination over him: an expression of privilege that others assert when they impose decisions concerning him that he disagrees with, prioritizing their aims and violating his will. There's a connection here, however offensive it may seem, between "breaking" and "gentling" horses with "breaking" and "gentling" my brother—between attitudes and practices that demand obedience and subordination to the sovereign will of others, and attitudes and practices rooted in fellow feeling and empathy that foster respect and self-respect.

Because of his TBI, Dan is more susceptible than most of us to being overcome by anger; triggering his anger requires less provocation, not only because his brain is scarred, but also because he has such limited control over so many aspects of his circumstances. Intentionally or not, Trinity Village's dealings with him—not reliably following schedules of care and ignoring his requests for help—underscored not only his own lack of control but also his reliance on staff members who were indifferent or even hostile toward him, forcing him to viscerally feel that reliance, which would have generated panic, mental (and sometimes physical) pain, and anger.

Conversely, Harbor's policy of allowing—even encouraging—residents to make decisions for themselves whenever possible helped Dan regain a sense of self-direction, of control over his own daily life. When one of his decisions somehow ran contrary to the facility's requirements for safety or to conformance to state and federal regulations, staff members worked to negotiate acceptable compromises. Additionally, the increased attention Dan received, attested to by daily shaves, physical and occupational therapy, and OBRA outings, reinforced his rightful claim that he matters.

As others exhibited a genuine concern for his wishes and respect for his person, he gained a greater degree of emotional flexibility. Acknowledging his right to autonomy and affirming his status of belonging within the Harbor community restored a more "normal" identity. His IED storms certainly didn't disappear, but they reduced in frequency and duration. As one Harbor attendant told me, it's not difficult and it doesn't take long to "talk him down."

The organic neurological effects of TBI are permanent, and so, also, is the survivor's susceptibility to resultant outbursts of anger. But progress is progress, and the progress Dan made at Harbor was remarkable.

★ ★ ★

A cadre of Harbor's physical and occupational therapists plunged into an enthusiastic partnership with Dan with the specific goal of helping him pass his June reassessment at Agape. Informed by Amy's list of goals and the photos and video clips I took during his initial assessment, the therapists generated a plan of action. It was ambitious and arduous, but both Dan and the therapy team were committed. Although their plan was geared toward improving Dan's ability to stay on a horse, the therapy would have other benefits as well. Strengthening his muscles (forearm, bicep, thigh, and core) and increasing flexibility in his hips would help him better balance his weight and sit more securely on a horse's back, but he would also be able to participate more in his transfers into and out of his wheelchair. Lifting and centering his head, which over years had developed a chronic pull downwards and to the right, would result in better riding posture, but it would also expand his field of vision and make swallowing (and therefore eating) easier.

Along with frequent therapy sessions involving stretching and strengthening exercises, Dan had taken it upon himself to begin maneuvering his wheelchair along Harbor's halls. These "walks" were extremely hard work, as he propelled the weight of the wheelchair as well as his own weight using only his left foot and leg. In the beginning, his progress along the hallways was painfully laborious and slow, but as the weeks passed, he gained in strength, comfort, and speed.

To open his hips enough to straddle a horse, Dan began wedging a ball between his knees from morning to night, even while making his daily rounds through the hallways. He began with a six-inch pliable plastic ball, only partly inflated but still demanding a challenging stretch from his stiffened hip joints and shortened muscles. Over the course of several months, he gradually increased the diameter of the balls, and by spring's end he was accommodating a fully inflated fifteen-inch ball with relative ease.

In early spring, Shiloh stopped me in the hallway as I was leaving Dan's room. "We're working on a surprise for Dan," she said. "I don't want to get his hopes up, in case it doesn't pan out, but I want to get your thoughts." Since Dan's appraisal at Agape, someone Shiloh knew had agreed to lend (and perhaps even donate) a saddle to Harbor's therapy department. Did I have any ideas for how therapists might use the saddle to help Dan accomplish his reassessment goals?

I recalled the wooden horse that Agape used in the initial stage of the assessment, which Dan had so vehemently objected to. We needed a different idea. I looked online for tools that riders use to maintain or increase their skills apart from the time they spend physically on a horse. I sent some images to Shiloh, who shared them with the therapists. Within a few weeks, one of the therapists constructed a wooden platform on wheels that braced a large plastic barrel topped with the saddle. A segment of each of Dan's therapy sessions now included sitting astride the barrel, helping him stretch the necessary muscles, tendons, and ligaments. After several weeks, the therapists began pushing the apparatus, first a few feet across the therapy room and then through the hallways, slowly increasing to a moderate speed, helping Dan gain strength and develop better balance.

The saddle-and-barrel contraption was therapeutically invaluable, supporting Dan's work on his motor skills, strength, and balance. But it was at least as useful in other ways, as well. The saddle was a tangible reminder (not that he would have forgotten) of the goal he was working toward, a symbol of something he had lost—an identity as much as an activity—presumably permanently, but now perhaps again within reach. And his increasing adeptness at accommodating the barrel marked his progress toward his ultimate goal. But just as importantly, whether consciously registered or not, it was irrefutable evidence that people at Harbor genuinely cared about him—that their concern extended beyond the baseline of keeping him alive. They were determined to help him tunnel into the region of rediscovered, deeply-held yearnings and aspirations, distinctive and horse-inflected, that gave renewed meaning to his life. Every time I saw that generous therapist's handiwork, my eyes watered with gratitude for the belonging it embodied—a belonging related, if not identical, to that purest form of love the ancient Greeks called *agape*.

★ ★ ★

In mid-February, Shiloh phoned me. She began with the nursing home mantra for nonemergency calls: "Don't be alarmed—everything's fine!" So often the reason she made phone calls to residents' families was to deliver unpleasant news, she told me, but this call was different; she wanted to update me on a positive development. Because the Indiana Friends van was for some reason unavailable for Dan's scheduled outing, Dan's attendant that day volunteered to transport him using her personal car so that he wouldn't miss his afternoon at the movies. Lacking the van's lift, she requested the help of Harbor personnel to get Dan into and out of her car, help that Shiloh and Adam, the director of nursing, offered. Dan rejected their assistance, of course, but he did allow them to stand nearby in case of trouble as he transferred himself from his wheelchair to Jenna's front seat. Shiloh just wanted to let me know that she'd been amazed by how well Dan had managed the transfer on his own that day—that his improvement was astonishing everyone who worked with him at Harbor. It had been rewarding for them all, she added, to see Dan achieve so much personal growth over the course of the year since he'd moved in, and they had recently noticed a drastic leap not only in his physical progress but also in terms of his enthusiasm and high spirits. Shiloh and I both agreed that the changes were likely due to Dan's reconnection to horses, which had revitalized him and inspired new goals. I don't doubt, however, that he was at least as uplifted by a new sense of social connection—of genuine belonging—he'd been missing for years.

Shiloh's call came on the heels of another encouraging conversation. The evening before, as I was leaving Harbor after a visit with Dan, his second-shift CNA pulled me aside in the hallway. Dan's personality, she said—especially his sense of humor, and the infectious smile and laughter that followed in its wake—had recently begun "shining through." He was pleasant, cheerful, more open, and friendlier with staff. He still had IED moments, she said, but there were fewer of them, and they were less disruptive (more easily defused, more quickly dissipated). Overall, he was bonding better with those who worked with him, and she wanted me to know how much happier he seemed.

Following these two conversations, I was downright giddy. I hadn't dared to formulate my goal for Dan so explicitly, but this—THIS— development was what I had so fervently hoped for.

★ ★ ★

Because I'm relating the real life of a TBI survivor in an effort (above all) to inform, rather than assembling a Hallmark Channel movie meant (above all) to inspire, I must emphasize that Dan's improvement, both physically and psychically, did not mean that his life suddenly had become smooth and trouble-free. My conversation with Shiloh took place on Monday; on my visit with Dan on Wednesday, we were passing through the dining hall when one of the physical therapists, Walter, stopped us to tell me that Dan had "wigged out" during their session that afternoon. Walter's disclosure had the air of tattling, a tone apparent to both Dan and me, so I wheeled Dan back to the privacy of his room before asking him what had happened.

He was forthcoming, as is his habit. First, shortly before Walter arrived at his room to pick him up for therapy, Dan had wet his pants—a chronic problem that I'd been urging him, unsuccessfully, to address ever since his arrival at Harbor—so he went to therapy in urine-soaked jeans, which embarrassed him and put him on edge. Adding to his aggravation, he believed that the towel-sliding exercise Walter had directed him to complete, because Dan found it too easy, constituted "busy work"—that it was a pro-forma exercise intended to burn therapy time. He was vexed by the thought that he was wasting precious therapy time instead of spending it constructively to work toward his goals. His IED kicked in, which Walter responded to by cutting their session short and whisking him back to his room. About an hour had passed when Walter, still clearly irritated with Dan, saw me and "told" on him.

Dan and I went together to the therapy department to tender an explanation, so that his therapists would not be left with the idea that he had "wigged out" for no reason. Walter had already left for the day, but therapists Darla and Kathy listened sympathetically as I explained Dan's mindset leading up to his outburst. Kathy assured Dan (and me) that she was well aware that he never exploded without some comprehensible reason—that there was always a discernible trigger for his storms. She also assured Dan that the towel-sliding exercise Walter had suggested was indeed useful—that it would help strengthen both his core and his shoulders.

Kathy and Darla were as warm, understanding, and accepting as I could have hoped for. I asked them to explain to Walter what had happened, because I believed he had taken Dan's outburst personally, and Dan hadn't intended to offend him.

After returning to his room, Dan and I discussed—for what seemed like the hundredth time—his incontinence problem. He insisted—also for the hundredth time—that he was *not* going to wear protective underwear (unfortunately referred to in common parlance as *adult diapers*, a term guaranteed to offend Dan and intensify his abhorrence of them). But this time, unlike my previous efforts to broach the conversation, the subject didn't tip Dan toward an IED event; in fact, he was remarkably unperturbed. He was adamant about not needing the pull-up underwear, but not angry. I took that as a sign of progress. He explained, again (but this time patiently, without the heat and anger that earlier discussions of the topic had consistently generated), that he was improving in so many ways that it was only a matter of weeks or—worst case scenario, possibly a few months—before he had this problem under control, too. I reminded him that when he arrived at Harbor the previous February, he'd been certain that his incontinence would no longer be an issue by September. It was now five months past that deadline, and there had been no signs of improvement. None. But there would be, he insisted—and soon, too.

The next morning when I called, Dan was in a great mood; he spelled "NEW" and "DRY" to let me know he was experiencing a new level of control regarding his drooling. He laughed with delight at his perceived progress, and also with happy anticipation of that afternoon's OBRA excursion. However, he called me a few hours later to tell me that he hadn't gone on the outing after all.

I was unable to piece together what had happened from Dan's responses on the phone, so I called the floor nurse, Marjorie, who related the whole episode. Dan had been ready to go, she said, and then at the last minute he had wet his pants. The Indiana Friends attendant told staff that if he wasn't changed and ready to go within five minutes, she was cancelling the outing. The nurse rushed to change his pants, but Dan had already become anxious and upset, which made the process more difficult and time-consuming. (He started to tip into a rage but managed to calm down when she told him she was going to walk out of his room if he pointed his middle finger at her.) Then there were last minute activities—putting on his coat, shutting off the TV, grabbing his letterboard—that apparently overtaxed the attendant's patience, who then left without him. So he didn't get his outing.

I had pleaded with Dan repeatedly, spurred by similar events, to agree to wearing pants protectors, if only on those days when he had an outing scheduled. If he were to improve to the point where he no longer wet his pants, I pledged, then he would have my blessing to stop using them, and I'd never say another word about it. Each time I made my case, when he didn't get angry, he shrugged, smiled, or laughed, and sometimes all three, but the conversation always ended with an emphatic shake of his head as he flatly refused to entertain the idea. He continued to insist that, because he sensed improvement in his drooling, he would spontaneously experience a corresponding improvement in continence. "But the two problems aren't related," I argued, trying to keep a tight rein on my exasperation. "The dynamics are different. Improving one issue doesn't affect the other. Your drooling is better because you've been working on holding your head up and lifting your chin. Wetting your pants is a completely unrelated problem. With one hand, it's still just as difficult to unzip your pants and position the urinal fast enough. It's entirely understandable that you'd have accidents; it would be hard for anyone. But that's why the protectors would be helpful."

No sale.

During one of these discussions, I noted with some aggravation, "I understand why you don't want to wear pants protectors. I really do. You think they'll mark you as more impaired than you really are, but they would actually have the opposite effect." I was aware that this subject was unavoidably delicate territory, and I was loath to compromise Dan's self-image or hurt his feelings—I don't want to do that, not *ever*—but it was my responsibility to help him fully grasp the reality that his refusal was constructing. I took a deep breath and continued, "It *matters* whether you go through your life in wet pants, smelling of urine, or not. It affects how people see you, how they think of you, how they treat you. Wetting your pants makes you smell bad, and it makes you look bad." The words stung my own mouth as they left it, but months of tip-toeing around these harsh realities had not helped him. It was up to me to drive home the dynamic, if I could. I went on. "How would it affect the way *you* thought of a guy if you saw him coming up the hall in a wheelchair with wet pants? How successfully independent would you think he was? What would you think of his level of mental competence?" Dan started to protest that urine-stained pants wouldn't make him think any less of that man, but my brother is, above all, honest. A slight sheepish smile played at his mouth and eyes as he realized that it would, indeed, lower his estimation of that person's mental capacity and self-control. As quickly as the thought came, however, he shrugged it off with a smile and shook his head as decisively as ever.

Anosognosia.

My point had landed, though—just not with the result I'd hoped for. In the days and weeks that followed this conversation, I would often find Dan with a paper napkin spread across his lap to conceal its dark stains.

At a care plan conference in November of 2019, the director of nursing, Adam, suggested that Dan take a medicine to help suppress urinary urgency. Long opposing any medicine, he flatly refused. But I continued to bring up the conversation every month or so, and sometimes more frequently as situations warranted. In May 2020, Dan insisted he was improving, so we negotiated another pact: if he could go two weeks without wetting his pants, he'd try the medicine. This time, he kept up his end of the bargain. Harbor ordered the medicine, and he took it faithfully without protest. Unfortunately, the drug didn't help, but I praised him for his flexibility. Maybe someday, I thought, he might agree to wear protective underwear, although when—and *if*—was still an open question.

★ ★ ★

From my journal, March 2, 2019:

> What really defines human beings for human beings? Our distinctive organizational cognitive and social/cultural patterns—the characteristic ways the human brain works that result, in effect, in *normal* human behavior. When there is a disruption to those patterns—whether cognitive, behavioral, or (especially) both—we view those who exhibit those disruptions as transgressive of human-ness—as less-than or otherly human.

For someone whose organizational patterns have been disrupted by TBI, the quest for acceptance as a fully relatable, fully human being is fraught with insult and degradation. Often, our lack of relatability to such people is steeped in a condescending kindness born of bewilderment—of coming face-to-face with someone who seems to occupy the liminal state of what we have learned to view as the not-quite-fully-human. Liminality is the space between boundaries, a position that straddles the line separating inclusion and exclusion from a given category. Liminality neither grants inclusion nor dictates exclusion; it indicates both/and, and neither/nor. Unless there are cultural practices or attitudes that help to normalize specific liminal spaces, someone who occupies one makes us uneasy, because they defy one or more of the relatively rigid categories we use to make sense of the world. When we don't know how to deal with the categorical straddler, we flail. And in that flailing, our reactions tend to reflect our confusion. Common responses are condescension, dismissal, and, worst of all, outright contempt.

It's this perplexity and its consequences that Dan points to when he bemoans others' tendency to treat him like a "BABY." The categorical confusion is understandable (but no less lamentable for that). Like babies, Dan can't speak. Like babies, he has what others view as "tantrums"—when an IED storm is triggered, he shouts and flails with anger, losing all emotional control. But he's not a baby; he is an adult man with problems. He has developed coping strategies that help him push through a barrage of challenges that the vast majority of people will never have to face. He's capable of adult interactions and relationships, when given the chance. At first blush, he straddles the organizational categories of both "baby" and "adult," and far too often others deal with him as a baby rather than as an adult, which of course offends his own sense of himself.

In our dealings with those people whose easy categorization is compromised by impaired functioning, we attempt to mask (even from ourselves) our discomfort, which arises from our difficulty in knowing how to firmly place such people in our world. We don't see how to offer them full acceptance as co-equal human beings, because they violate at least some of the attributes we associate with humanness (e.g., language use and socially acceptable levels of self-control and autonomy). We sense that their call is for social identification and belongingness, and if we are unequipped to answer it, we are unsettled. Without experiences that have trained us to recognize these people's just claim to full membership in the human community, we're likely to respond with confoundment, fear, anxiety, anger, or even disgust (a reaction to something or someone deemed categorically out of place). The problem is, only our heartfelt acceptance of our fellow human beings—including those who are unable to consistently demonstrate what our social expectations demand for "normal" behavior or appearance, for whatever reason—can make them (or us) feel any better.

There is an effective and fully realizable answer: we can create a new category for people who are cognitively, neurologically, physically, and/or socially impaired, a category that transcends the normative attributes we have historically insisted upon for full inclusion. We can acknowledge that someone's thoughts and behavior may not always follow our expectations without summarily rejecting their full humanity, by recognizing the already-existent ground of differently functioning but still fully human being. Such a recognition requires only the understanding that, at core, neither our genetic makeup nor our ability to conform to established patterns is what makes us human. Rather, the ground upon which our humanity rests is our essential need for human acceptance. While other species may benefit from belonging to and within the human community, for human beings this belongingness is a fundamental matter of psychic, and often physical, survival. We can't live truly human lives without it.

★ ★ ★

In the first week in February, I got a call from Dan's nurse Marjorie again. "Dan fell," she said, quickly adding, "but he wasn't hurt." Because of a staff shortage that day, the morning CNA was late getting to his room to get him out of bed and dressed. Impatient and angry at the delay, Marjorie said, he decided he would get up by himself, which consequently led to a fall. Because he had fallen, staff was required to take his vital signs, but when they tried, she said, Dan "pitched a fit."

It wasn't until several days later that I learned that Dan had not fallen. Because of his intensive work with physical and occupational therapists in preparation for the horseback riding, he told me, he decided to test his ability to transfer into his wheelchair unassisted. Using his newly developed strength, core control, and balance, he carefully slid down from the bed to the floor, intending to pull himself into the chair. He was painstakingly working on the transfer when a CNA entered the room before he'd had a chance to complete the maneuver. The CNA assumed that Dan had been enraged at the disruption in his schedule and consequently had lost all control, essentially hurling himself out of bed onto the floor. Alarmed, the CNA fussed over him, checking for injuries, while she scolded him for his impatience. Dan felt profoundly misunderstood: he hadn't been either angry or foolhardy; he was cautiously testing the extent of his redeveloping skills. Since he hadn't fallen, he saw no reason for their alarm and chastisement, and no need for them to take his vitals. The combination of the assumption that he'd been short-tempered and querulous, the scolding that had followed, and what he saw as overprotectiveness arising from underestimating his abilities, resulted in an all-but-inevitable IED storm.

When we discussed the episode four days later, Dan was completely receptive to my presentation of Harbor's perspective. He agreed that the conclusion staff had drawn when they walked into the room and found him on the floor was a reasonable one. He saw that they were just doing their jobs as responsibly as they could. He spelled "VERY THANK," asking me to convey his thanks to the staff for their conscientious concern and care. I did, and they were as pleased by Dan's apology for his outburst as they were surprised by his explanation of the event.

The same day, I also corrected the record with Adam. We not only discussed the one specific transfer event, but we talked more generally about Dan's and his family's perspective that Dan himself is responsible for the decisions he makes. I pledged that, while we certainly hoped that none of his decisions would lead to injury, we would not hold Harbor liable if one did. Adam noted that if any such event occurred, Harbor would have to file a report with the state in accordance with accountability requirements, and I offered that I'd be willing to attest to Dan's and our position to whatever negligence authorities might suspect of Harbor. I understood, even as I tendered that pledge, that Harbor would not be legally protected by it—that, in that situation, they would have nothing more to count on than my word to hold them blameless. Nor did I want to consider a blanket waiver that would free Harbor of accountability in case any of their employees did, in fact, exercise negligence or poor judgment that resulted in harm to Dan. Certainly, we would never pursue a complaint without evidence of real wrongdoing, but neither would we let evidence of wrongdoing go unexplored. As a matter of fact, just the previous week I had filed a complaint against Trinity Village with Georgia state authorities, which Harbor administrators were aware of. I assured Adam that Dan, Dave, and I were not prone to legal action, and I didn't believe we would ever regard Harbor the same way we viewed

Trinity Village. Trinity Village had a crossed line, and done real harm to my brother, with the administration of drugs that were not only unnecessary but also inappropriate and often dangerous to someone in Dan's position. (Although nothing more than an investigation ever came from my complaint, I'm still glad I filed it—not only because Dan wanted me to, but also because I would have felt as though I had neglected a serious responsibility to [at least attempt to] hold accountable those who had abused Dan's and his family's trust, and to try to prevent other Trinity Village residents from suffering the same treatment.)

At this juncture of the conversation, Adam noted that Dan (now medication-free for eighteen months) was seldom experiencing behavioral issues and that when he did have an IED event, it quickly passed. I noted that the triggers for his outbursts were typically identifiable: he feels like he's being pushed to do something he doesn't want to do, prevented from doing something he does want to do, or feels he's being overlooked or underestimated (which includes instances when people are making what he considers to be an unnecessary fuss over him). The antidote to his outbursts were equally identifiable: reassure him through personal interactions that he is viewed as a competent adult who has the right to make his own decisions, as long as those decisions don't endanger anyone else. Adam smiled and nodded. I agreed that the outbursts were certainly unpleasant when they occurred, but I also noted that I firmly believe that without the attitude that activates them, Dan surely would have died a long time ago—that his persistent drive for independence and dignity had kept him alive, as he pushed his way with sheer force of will through some monumental obstacles in some very dark times.

Adam nodded, adding, "We'll take it."

★ ★ ★

At the end of April, about five weeks before Dan's scheduled re-evaluation at Agape, Harbor arranged a horseback riding outing for Dan—a sort of practice run to see where he was in terms of his progress. One aim was to uncover any remaining deficits that would prevent him from being accepted into Agape's program, so that therapists could fine-tune their rehabilitative efforts in the final stretch before his reassessment. Another aim was to provide footage for a five-minute publicity video for Harbor. After all Harbor had done to improve Dan's life, not least of all orchestrating such inspiring and innovative efforts to ready him for his riding reassessment, Dan and I were happy to participate in any project that promoted the facility.

So on April 23, Dan and I assembled with Harbor administrators and therapists at the Henry County Saddle Club in New Castle, about half an hour away from Muncie, for an afternoon trial ride. The regional director of Harbor and his wife were already waiting for us, along with Scout, one of eleven horses they owned, and their daughter Sammi, who had spent weeks training Scout in preparation for Dan's ride. (Sammi was planning a career as a hippotherapist, and this event was the culmination and a test of her efforts to prepare both herself and her horse for that work.) Shiloh met us there, along with Adam—not only Harbor's director of nursing but also the owner of the racehorse whose framed poster decorated a wall in Dan's room—and therapists Annie, Darla, and Kathy. Ian, the professional photographer, videographer, and marketing specialist for the corporation that owns Harbor Health, was already set up to film our arrival, as well as the ride itself.

As Dan rode Scout, I took video with my phone to share afterward with the therapy team, as well as to send to Dave so he could share in Dan's ride and his post-ride interactions with Scout. My photos and clips paled in comparison to the striking fifty-one-second trailer Ian completed that night for the finished video, which would be assembled in the coming days for release several weeks later.

The day after Dan's ride, Ian held a series of interviews at Harbor in a pleasant, sun-drenched lounge. I was interviewed first, and then I sat with Dan just off-camera as Shiloh and therapists Darla, Annie, and Kathy answered questions about their experiences working with him. I was profoundly moved as this cadre of smart, caring women expressed their obvious personal as well as professional interest in my brother, and I was grateful that Dan was present to hear it. They interacted with him on an ongoing and periodically daily basis, so they genuinely knew him, which was key to the significance of their appreciation of him and their affection for him. When during her interview Darla tearfully observed, "Dan is an awesome person," a penetrating warmth radiated through me. Dan surely felt it too, only tenfold, as the channels that connected him to others—channels that had long lain parched and barren—flooded with belongingness.

★ ★ ★

Just prior to his reassessment for acceptance into Agape's program, Dan experienced an increase in IED storms. As I wrote in my journal at the end of May,

> The road is never smooth. . . . As the time for him to start at Agape (next Monday, six days from now) nears, it seems to have upped his emotional level, so that it's perhaps decreasing the threshold required to trigger an IED event.

I noted that, in my reading, I had come across a counseling tool called CBT, which sometimes proves helpful to TBI survivors who are trying to reduce their struggles with IED. The idea behind the therapy is simple: we don't react to events; we react to the way we *think* about events. By changing our thinking about events, we can change the way we react to them.

I talked to Dan about this practice and told him that, if he were interested in pursuing this avenue, I would try to learn more about it, and we could tackle the IED together. He was surprisingly receptive to the idea. As I continued in my journal, "It's the first time I know of that he has acknowledged IED as a problem he'd like to work on, rather than just a dismissible aspect of who he is now. I think he's become more aware of his social image and how much better social inclusion feels. . . . This new openness may seem insignificant to anyone who hasn't known him for the past four decades, but it's genuinely big. And promising. I hope I can help."

★ ★ ★

On June 3, Amy and her staff re-assessed Dan's capabilities to participate in Agape's riding program. The half-hour flew by. As he exchanged a post-ride snuggle with Bo, the friendly and healthy but aged Appaloosa who had been assigned as his riding partner, both Dan and I glowed under Amy's praise. The progress he'd made since January, she said, was nothing short of astonishing. "He's worked really hard in therapy," I noted, to which she replied, "And it shows!"

To someone who hadn't carefully evaluated his performances both in January and in June, the degree of improvement Dan had reached would not have been evident. He was still unable to sit unsupported on Bo's back, and his hips still lacked the flexibility to allow his legs to drape fully over Bo's ribs. He still required frequent readjustment to accommodate slippage from side to side. But his grip on the pommel was steely, his knees no longer hovered above Bo's neck, and he better accommodated Bo's swaying as they moved around the arena.

Halfway through the assessment, Dan spelled, "GALLOP."

Amy and her raft of volunteers laughed. "Maybe not quite yet, Dan," Amy said.

Dan was accepted into Agape's program that day. He would have half-hour lessons once a week. When we arrived back at Harbor, he told me he wanted hour-long lessons, and I told him that if he wanted to increase the duration later, as he built up his strength, flexibility, balance, and conditioning, we could likely arrange it. But half an hour, for the time being, was likely a good start.

Given his soreness the next day, Dan agreed. But despite the aches, there was a new luminescence in his eyes, a brightness that I was sure I'd seen there before, but I couldn't quite remember when. Within a week, he asked me to help him order a new riding helmet. We scanned several websites before purchasing a handsome new Charles Owen helmet with a blue Lycra cover, emblazoned on the back with his initials in white: DH.

Dan Hicks was back in the saddle.

Notes

1. Omnibus Budget Reconciliation Act of 1987, 100th Congress, Pub.L. 100–203, 101 Stat. 1330–160, Title IV(C), Sec. 1819 (B) (2). https://budgetcounsel.files.wordpress.com/2017/01/omnibus-budget-reconciliation-act-of-1987.pdf
2. Omnibus Budget Reconciliation Act of 1987, Sec. 1819 (B) (1) (A).
3. Omnibus Budget Reconciliation Act of 1987, Sec. 1819 (c) (1) (a) (ii).
4. Lawrence Scanlan, "The Gentle Art of the Horse Whisperer," in *Wild About Horses: Our Timeless Passion for the Horse* (New York: HarperCollins, 2001), 84–117.

9   Newer Normal

Summer 2019 was a banner period for Dan. He was revitalized by his revived involvement with horses. Not only had OBRA, Harbor Health, and Agape provided him with the opportunity to sit astride a horse again, which was helping him regain some of the strength and balance he'd lost over the years, but also his reconnection to horses and to equicentric culture was restoring a hefty measure of his pre-accident identity and some of the spiritual equilibrium that went with it. Earlier in the year, the prospect of immersing himself again in the world of horses had given him new goals, which he pursued with vigor. He built up his strength and endurance by working hard in therapy, and by propelling himself through the building's hallways for hours each day, one foot-push at a time, proudly reporting on our bedtime phone calls the number of laps he'd completed on that day's "walks." Over the previous three decades Dan had formed the habit of watching TV every waking hour, but he had begun allowing the screen to remain black and silent until bedtime. He asked me to bring him a radio, and what little time Dan passed in his room, he now mostly spent listening to a local country station as he watched birds flitting in the courtyard and devouring seed at his window. Reacquainted with his appreciation for country music, he soon recognized the voices and songs of contemporary balladeers, and while they could never replace Waylon and Willie in his esteem, he enjoyed their contributions to his days and evenings.

Dan's long-ingrained routine was changing in another, even startling, way, which I discovered one afternoon when I arrived at Harbor for an unscheduled visit. Walking toward his room, I caught sight of my brother in the communal dining hall, seated at one of the tables. I changed course to draw nearer. Harbor was hosting its monthly Happy Hour gathering, and a local musician was strumming a guitar and singing to a karaoke version of "Margaritaville," as a dozen or so residents—Dan one of them—snacked from small paper plates bearing tortilla chips, salsa, and barbecued cocktail wieners.

Dan's presence at such a function astonished me. Over the years, he had increasingly and at some point consistently, even vehemently, refused to engage in resident activities. He had preferred instead the isolation of his room, where he kept his psychological as well as physical distance from other residents, who were overwhelmingly elderly and cognitively tenuous. Not surprisingly, Dan didn't view them as his peers. In his social seclusion, he could experience himself as more "normal"—younger, more mentally vigorous, grounded, and alert—than the dementia patients who stared aimlessly or nodded off in the hallways, or who jabbered nonsense into the air. Dan had formed the habit of keeping to himself, determined not to identify, or to be identified by others, with those surrounding him. It was a population he had little in common with, except for their need for assistance in accomplishing essential daily tasks related to dressing, personal hygiene, mobility, and toileting—not a characteristic he wanted to focus on in himself. So even though Dan sat alone at his table as he munched chips and listened to covers of 1970s pop songs, his very presence in Margaritaville signaled a departure from his longstanding customary inclination to keep to himself.

Other surprises began emerging at the same time. Instead of eating his meals from a tray alone in his room, Dan began taking breakfast, lunch, and dinner in the dining hall. He established his own place at a table with Sam, a man in his seventies with rapidly advancing Parkinson's disease and dementia, and Sam's wife Larue, who was sociable, kind, and neighborly to Dan. The fourth seat at their table was sporadically filled by residents who rotated positions from time to time, but Sam, Larue, and Dan formed a reliable threesome each day. Larue chatted amiably with Dan and quickly learned his mealtime preferences, relaying and clarifying them to recent hires who weren't yet familiar with Dan's modus operandi. Dan liked eating with Sam and Larue and now preferred the bustle of the dining hall to taking meals in his room with only the radio or television for company.

Along with attending Happy Hours and eating in the dining hall, Dan began scanning Harbor's monthly activities calendar. Every Wednesday, activities staff offered an expedition for residents, with trips ranging from shopping at Walmart or lunch at a local eatery to special excursions such as Special Olympics competitions or afternoons at the zoo in Ft. Wayne. Wheelchair seating on the bus was limited, and seats for the special trips went quickly—too quickly for us to secure a place for Dan by the time he decided whether or not he wanted to go—but there was less participation in local lunches. While Dan had no interest in shopping at Walmart (despite the Subway sandwiches that followed), he occasionally asked me to sign him up for a restaurant trip. The food was seldom anything special, and he sometimes found these activities boring, but since he'd begun participating in OBRA excursions, he had come to appreciate changes in routine and scenery, even in the company of other residents he felt little connection to.

The frequency of our phone calls also dramatically changed. For the first eighteen months that Dan lived at Harbor, I called him every morning and every night, just to check in—to see how his day was going, to make sure that I knew of any issues that needed attention or interventions he wanted me to make on his behalf. He often called me sporadically throughout the day, either to alert me to some problem he was encountering or just to touch base. By midsummer, though, he seldom called during the day, and he rarely answered the phone when I called in the morning, because he wasn't in his room. For most of the day, he was too busy socializing, exercising, or participating in OBRA or Harbor outings to answer my calls. I gradually stopped calling him except before bedtime, trusting that all was well during the day unless I heard from him. And it always was.

So by the end of summer, Dan was no longer cloistered in his room from morning to night, passively watching reruns of old football games or movies he'd already seen too many times. Instead, he was exercising his body and cultivating his long-neglected sociality, exchanging frequent greetings with staff and a select few residents as he wheeled through the hallways and participated in residential activities. Even when he was not receiving physical therapy, each day his walks took him to Harbor's therapy department, where the therapists amiably welcomed him, chatting and joking with him as their work duties allowed. His weeks were structured by his three OBRA excursions—most importantly, the rides with Bo at Agape—and occasionally supplemented by one of Harbor's lunch outings. And three times a day, every day, he was taking his meals in the dining hall, keeping company with Sam and Larue and whomever else he encountered as he ate.

I think it's no coincidence that Dan's dramatic shift from social withdrawal to bustling sociality followed directly on the heels of his re-engagement with horses and riding culture. Recapturing his own identity as a horseman—a special figure in a rarified world—enabled him to associate with others in the nursing home community in which he lived. He was a horseman again—and, perhaps just as importantly, those around him knew it. He possessed a unique identity within Harbor, not only because he was younger and brain-injured rather than elderly and failing in the final months or last few years of life but because he now owned both a past and a present that connected him to horses.

This uniqueness he treasured. It was a uniqueness honored—grasped, respected, and frequently referred to—by others. No longer plagued by the ghost of his lost identity, and now clearly differentiated from those suffering a dementia-ridden old age, Dan was voluntarily engaging in activities that brought him pleasure, even if that pleasure was as modest as tortilla chips, salsa, cocktail wieners, and a rousing medley of Jimmy Buffet songs.

★ ★ ★

On one of our phone calls shortly after he began his lessons at Agape in June, Dan spelled, "HORSES RACE" and "INDIANA." He had heard a radio ad for the Indiana Grand, a bustling racetrack and casino about a 1-1/2-hour drive from Muncie. On the outskirts of the relatively rural town of Shelbyville, I had never heard of the place. But the ad touted the venue's hosting of the Indiana Derby in mid-July. And he fervently wished to go.

I had never been to a racetrack, nor had I ever wanted to go to one. I had read a number of nonfiction books about horse racing to Dan, but only to indulge his passion for it. I myself have objected to racing for decades, when I first became aware of (and then more informed about) the innumerable abuses that our culture inflicts on animals. I'm unequivocally opposed to practices that use animals for human convenience or indulgence—any purpose, really, that conflicts with the animals' own well-being—and that certainly includes horse racing.

Still, when Dan excitedly told me that there was a racetrack relatively close to us in Muncie, and that it was hosting a Derby Day the following month, I decided that, while I would have to check with Dyke before making any promises, I would try to get him to it. And as I suspected would be the case, Dyke agreed to the plan—his assent always an act of generosity, since I'm of limited use with the heavy lifting required to take Dan out in the absence of a van with a lift. It would be Dyke who would help Dan in and out of our car, lift the wheelchair into and out of our trunk, buddy-walk Dan to and from his seat at the track, and escort him to the bathroom as necessary.

Once it was a fact that we were going, I was a bit nervous for all of us regarding the logistics: taking Dan to an unfamiliar place, making our way around the facility, finding a seat for him that was accessible and comfortable but that still provided a good view of the track, and working out the details of his eating a meal without the convenience of a table to hold food and drinks. However, despite these issues, and even though my conscience grated at the idea of patronizing a racetrack, I was glad to help

Dan experience something that mattered so much to him. Taking him to the races was exactly as morally problematic for Dyke and me as it is when we treat him to a cheeseburger, burrito, or pizza every Sunday. Even though we've both been vegetarian for over thirty years, Dan is not, and buying his animal-laden lunches doesn't really constitute a dilemma for us. We treat him to lunch; he is free, as is everyone else we know, to select the meals he wants for himself. In the same way, left to our own devices, Dyke and I would never attend a horse race. But we gladly agreed to take Dan to Shelbyville for the special outing that he had so fervently chosen.

When I told him we definitely were going to the Indiana Derby, Dan added another request: he wanted to visit the backstretch, the area apart from the racetrack where the horses, grooms, jockeys, and others associated with track life live and loiter before and after their races. I promised that I would try to arrange a visit, but I doubted that the public was allowed behind the scenes. Dan insisted that I was mistaken; in his time as a groom at Los Alamitos, spectators visited the backstretch all the time. I would look into it, I told him.

I phoned the Indiana Grand several weeks before Derby Day. I briefly explained Dan's situation—his history with horse racing and the accident that suddenly disrupted his pursuit of his passion for all things horses and racing—and what we were hoping to arrange—to a helpful, warmhearted woman named June. She described in detail the layout of the various seating areas, which gave me at least a vague sense of how we might negotiate the logistics. She was truly sorry, she said, but the backstretch was closed to the public. Years before there had been few restrictions on access to such areas, but an increase in sabotage had been met with tightened security. Because of the risk of owners or trainers hiring henchmen to illicitly drug or even maim their competitors' horses, or to approach jockeys with bribes to throw races or trainers to fix them, the public was now barred from any area where they might encounter horses or workers beyond the watchful eye of officials. Unless we had a personal connection to someone who worked in the backstretch and so would vouch for us, June said, we would be limited to public areas for viewing and betting.

Dan was disappointed that we wouldn't be mingling with the horses and personnel behind the scenes in the backstretch, but he was thrilled by the prospect of attending Derby Day itself. Several times on our phone calls and visits in the weeks leading up to our outing, Dan spelled, "VERY THANKS HORSE."

Despite my trepidation, I was looking forward to the event on Dan's behalf, and it went as well as I could have hoped. We first explored the seating available on a long patio between the racetrack building and the track, but we chose to move indoors, out of the midsummer heat.

Having visited racetracks only in my imagination as shaped by the books I'd read to Dan, I had imagined the facility would be somewhat seedy, but the Indiana Grand was bright, modern, well-kept, and even a bit ritzy—a study in muted earth-toned fabrics, spotless carpeting and shiny tile floors, and well-polished chrome. The elevators were spacious, and they gently lifted us to the second floor, where we found a tiered bank of theater seats facing a glass wall. It provided a broad view of the entire track and much of the bright blue sky above it, so that's where we settled. Some spirited attendees had dressed up in Derby tradition, sporting tuxedos and top hats or fancy gossamer-and-lace dresses, elbow-length gloves, and hats swirled with feathers, flowers, and veils. Suddenly June appeared at Dan's elbow, having recognized us from my phone conversation with her, and introduced herself. She handed Dan a program containing the racing schedule and information about the horses and jockeys, along with a commemorative Indiana Derby lapel pin. June's warm welcome set reinforced Dan's sense of broad social connection, based sheerly on shared interests, to strangers who surround us at events we attend.

We had arrived early enough that we had our choice of seats, so we commandeered three on an aisle four rows from the top, enabling quick trips to the betting windows, the soda counter, and the bathrooms. I spent much of the afternoon drifting from one to the other, preferring to remain in motion so that I had less time to consider what was required to get those horses to run so hard. Fortunately, that afternoon, none of them were carted off the track due to fractured bones, torn ligaments, or any of the other injuries that befall these animals during races. But knowing that injury and death are continual threats to these animals, I hustled drinks and placed Dan's bets in an effort not to think about it.

The Derby excursion went so well that the next month, when Dave was in town for a visit, the four of us went to the Indiana Grand for a day of quarter horse racing, Dan's particular interest. Dan wanted to sit closer to the window than we had at the Derby, to feel the action more vividly. Because there were no wheelchair ramps, Dave buddy-walked him down twenty or thirty steps—no easy feat, even for Dave, still strong and athletic but now in his mid-sixties. At one point, I accidentally kicked over Dan's twenty-four-ounce cup of chocolate milk, soaking the otherwise spotless carpet, and so made countless trips back and forth to the bathroom for rafts of wet, soapy paper towels to clean up the mess. And sadly, the equine ambulance carried away a downed horse from the track following his (very likely last) race. On this trip, we stayed at the track late into the evening, so that all of us were exhausted by the time we got back to Harbor.

Because he was so tired, rather than wait for a CNA to help him to bed, Dan insisted that we do it. But by this time, I was fatigued, and out of sorts. I just wanted to go home and felt that Dan's refusal to wait for the CNA was inconsiderate and unnecessarily burdensome. When I declared that I was done for the day, Dan (who was also completely worn out) flew into an IED storm—flailing, hollering, and energetically brandishing his middle finger specifically at me.

Although I know with utter certainty that Dan's rages are beyond his control, his outburst triggered one of my own. Although mine was quieter and more bounded, it was almost as vehement. After the day I'd had—running Dan's bets, standing in slow lines to buy his drinks and nachos, mopping up chocolate milk, cleaning him up after his refreshments, and watching a beautiful suffering animal carted off to likely slaughter—Dan's contorted face and waving middle finger struck me as utterly unjust and maddeningly unappreciative. "Oh, so I haven't done enough for you today?" I snarled, equally churlish.

In the end, I stood aside in resentful turmoil as Dave and Dyke helped Dan undress and get into bed. I think—but I'm not certain—I wished him a good night before leaving.

The next day, I recounted my sense of the episode in my journal:

> What that finger means: I don't like you; I don't care about you; fuck you. What *I* want is the only thing that matters—*you* don't matter, other than in terms of what you do for me.
>
> Dan's finger, his outbursts, are painful to the recipient, but they're also counterproductive for him. It's hard to remember that he's expressing a feeling that's only true in the moment. I fear that people who aren't necessarily invested in him and on the receiving end of that fury will find it hard to like him; to the degree they can, people will avoid him; they'll do the bare minimum for him, and resent having to do that.
>
> It's sad—I'm his sister, and still, that's all it took for me. I know better, and yet, in those moments, I felt used and despised.
>
> Even loving Dan as I do, and even knowing that IED is a neurological disorder he can't control, it's hard for me to manage the feelings that arise under that kind of ugly assault. *Everyone* needs acceptance and belonging—no one is immune to the pain of feeling rejected by someone they care about. That includes me. I need to belong to Dan as much as he needs to belong to me. That's what got me so upset: faced with his fury, I felt the moorings of belongingness slip.
>
> Family members have problems and issues that have nothing to do with the TBI survivor—that he is neither responsible for nor

able to resolve. The survivor isn't—and shouldn't necessarily be—at the center of others' lives at all times. That asks too much of everyone; it compromises both the survivor's and the family member's or caregiver's sense of discrete identity. Belonging can't be imposed by chains. It's a product of caring, not compulsion.

It's a complex problem, hard to negotiate and impossible to solve, even when family members are well-intentioned and try their best. Being aware of belongingness issues and helping to increase belongingness can help make things better, but TBI is an inevitably difficult condition for survivors, their families, and their caregivers. It feels, because it is, intractable.

But, while the problem can't be solved, it can be accepted and endured, if only because Dan's human, and so am I. I forgive him for his outbursts, and I should forgive my own lapses with equal sympathy.

Pretty good advice.

Several weeks later, I added, "True enough, the survivor shouldn't necessarily be the center of everyone's lives *all the time*—but one of the essential aspects of belongingness is that the person must know that he does, in times of genuine need, come first in at least *someone's* life."

Also pretty good advice.

★ ★ ★

Toward the end of September, I received an email from the program director for the local office of Indiana Friends, the service that provided staff for Dan's OBRA outings. I had been gratefully impressed by Indiana Friends's services. Ella, the assistant who was usually assigned to all three of Dan's weekly excursions, was in her mid-thirties and struck me as kind, energetic, and dependable, and she communicated with Dan in a spirit that conveyed equality and friendly respect. In fact, she was even learning the manual alphabet so that she could better understand him.

On the rare outing days when Ella was assigned elsewhere, Starr was designated to fill in for her. Starr was barely out of her teens and yet seemed even younger. She sped the Indiana Friends van down the rural roads toward Agape, heedless of how the ride jostled her passengers. The violent bouncing caused Dan to slide down in his wheelchair, leaving him nearly horizontal on his back, and unable to reposition himself. Also, even though her job required that she closely interact with Dan, often with a considerable degree of physical intimacy, she dressed in thin shirts and strategically torn jeans that fit her like skin. She flitted around Dan, playfully poking him in the ribs or belly, teasing him about how "cute" he was and how much he "liked" her. I tried not to be overly judgmental of her coquetry or her suggestive style of dress; I remembered (if only distantly) my own adolescent discovery that sexual allure was a newly available form of power, with force and boundaries I myself had tested in ways that were likely out of line at times. I was uneasy about how Dan might respond to her provocative behavior, but I was more concerned about the discomfort and potential safety risks she subjected him to with her incautious driving. Dan, for his part, was fond of Ella, who treated him like an adult she both liked and respected, but he wasn't drawn to Starr and her schoolgirl flirtations, which struck him as silly and condescending (as indeed they were). He took her in stride as she fluttered about, simply appreciative that, even on those days when Ella was unavailable, he could still go to Agape, lunch, or the movies.

Then, in September, a shoe dropped. Helen, the supervisor of Dan's Indiana Friend's attendants, sent me an email that began, "I think we have an issue that we need to work through." Ella, she said, had reported that Dan had "been inappropriate with her" in ways she had initially interpreted as accidental. However, the day before, there was no mistaking his intentionality; he had placed his hand on Ella's breast and laughed. Ella wondered if Dan had misunderstood the nature of their relationship, but whatever the reason for his behavior, she was shocked and affronted by it, and she no longer wanted to work with him. When Helen asked Starr if she would take Ella's place as Dan's primary assistant, she refused, saying that she wasn't comfortable around him because he had inappropriately touched her, too. Helen tentatively added that Ella had expressed her possible willingness to keep working with Dan if he apologized and if she felt confident that he would never repeat the behavior.

I was aghast. I was certainly upset on behalf of the women, but I also knew what this complication might mean for Dan: the discontinuation of the outings that had so revitalized him. I went to Harbor that afternoon, mindful that berating him would accomplish nothing constructive—in fact, would be counterproductive. The situation called for a chance for Dan to explain himself and, most importantly, learn from. I read the director's email to Dan and asked him if it was accurate. He nodded, then ducked his head and covered his eyes with his hand—his gesture for embarrassment and remorse.

We discussed the problem for quite some time. In response to my questions, Dan relayed that he hadn't misinterpreted his relationship with Ella, but he had hoped that when he expressed his sexual interest, she might return it. I asked him if he had ever touched any other woman without her assent, and he nodded. I asked him if any woman had ever responded positively to his unsolicited advances, and he met my gaze ruefully, shook his head, and again covered his eyes, abashed. He assured me that he understood that this behavior wasn't just counterproductive to his own interests, but it was also transgressive, an offense to the women whose boundaries he'd trespassed. I told him that, as someone who'd been subjected to similar behavior more than once when I was younger, I could verify that this kind of boundary-crossing is deeply upsetting, hoping that connecting such behavior to its effects on his own sister might drive the lesson home. I also told him that I was sorrier than I could say (and in fact I was near tears when I said it), but he had to know that one of the many things his accident had taken from him was the possibility of courtship, romantic love, and sexual bonding. It pained me to the core to point it out, I said, but Dan needed to acknowledge that harsh reality, so that he wouldn't make the same mistake again. He looked gravely into my eyes and nodded.

A few hours later, I responded to Helen's email, assuming that she would share its contents with Ella and Starr. I wrote,

> I did talk to Dan. He is as embarrassed as he is sorry. He realizes his actions were indeed inappropriate, and he does want to apologize to both Ella and Starr, and he pledges never, ever to do it again. He didn't misunderstand their relationship; he was hoping (but not expecting) that they might have some sexual interest in him, and he's very embarrassed by that.
>
> (Please note: This next paragraph is all me; it doesn't come from Dan.) I would not ask or expect either Ella or Starr to excuse his inappropriate behavior—it was wrong and totally merits an apology, as well as his promise never to repeat it—but I would like to point out that his accident happened when he was eighteen years old.... He has been completely left out of the world of romance, dating, and sex. While the accident pretty completely erased any chance that he would have romantic sexual relationships with women, it didn't diminish his interest in them.
>
> Dan understands that his advances were unwarranted and unwelcome, and he would like to apologize to Ella and Starr in person and let them know that that behavior will *not* be repeated....

A few days later, Ella, Starr, and I met with Dan in his room. Ella explained to him at length that she had felt disrespected by his actions, which had given her no say in when she was touched, where, or by whom. Dan listened quietly, intently, and then he apologized, assuring her (through me) that he never meant to convey disrespect; he liked her very much and did indeed respect her. Ella thanked him for his apology and accepted it. Although she would make no promises now, she said, she would consider working with him again, as she trusted that he was sincere.

Dan apologized to Starr, too. She said that the day after he had grabbed her bottom, they had gone to Pizza King for lunch, where he had spelled "SONABITCH" on his Speak'n'Spell. She had assumed he was angry at her, she said, for not responding positively to his advances. He shook his head. "NO. SORRY," he spelled.

After the women had left, I told Dan I was proud of him. He had taken responsibility for his behavior, sincerely apologized for it, and pledged not to repeat it. More could not be asked of him or done by him, other than that he follow through on his promise. We would just have to see how things shook out and hope for the best. I was surprised, however, to discover that, while he clearly remembered and acknowledged his offense against Ella, he had no memory of inappropriately touching Starr. He had apologized to her because she claimed he had violated her boundaries, so he assumed that he must have brushed against her accidentally, without knowing it.

The next day, Ella phoned me, mainly in response to Starr's reference to the Pizza King outing, which had taken place five weeks earlier. At the time, I had received an email from Helen, requesting that I "do some investigating" for her. On his lunch excursion to Pizza King with Starr that day, the email explained, Dan had gotten "upset" and spelled "son bit★★" on his Speak'n'Spell. Helen noted that Starr "was clueless as to why he was upset . . . she honestly wasn't sure what happened," so Helen asked me to talk to Dan, to find out why he'd been angry.

I asked Dan about the episode the same day I got Helen's email. He couldn't find the words to explain what had distressed him; he said only that Starr didn't like him. Then he indicated that he wanted to drop the subject and asked me not to bring it up again. I told him that Starr was scheduled to take him to Agape the next day; was that a problem for him? "NO." When he returned from Agape the following day, I asked him if the excursion had gone okay, and he said "YES." It seemed to me that whatever the problem had been, it had been resolved. I wrote to Helen to let her know and to thank her for her concern.

But when Ella phoned me the day after Dan's apology, I gained insight into the conflict between Starr and Dan. When Ella took Dan to Pizza King the week after Starr had, the restaurant manager called her aside. The week before, the manager told her, she'd received complaints from three different customers, conveyed through the waitress who had served Dan, about Starr and a coworker who had accompanied her. The customers had been distressed because Starr and the other assistant were "belittling"

Dan, taunting him to the point that those at the tables around them were uncomfortable. One customer complained that Starr and her coworker had had emptied Dan's urinal in the restaurant parking lot, and then left Dan sitting alone in his wheelchair outside the van, on unshaded asphalt in August, while they smoked cigarettes and chatted under a tree on a distant corner of the lot. Leaving Dan unattended constituted a breach of Indiana Friends's safety regulations, and emptying his urinal in such a setting violated public health standards, but both acts were especially egregious to me for the message they sent to Dan about his relational status. Paired with the derision he'd been subjected to in the restaurant, their message was one of unmistakable contempt.

Ella told me that she'd reported the restaurant manager's concerns to Helen. But Helen, as the director of a program constantly facing the threat of inadequate staffing, hadn't even questioned Starr or her coworker about the incident. Apparently, Helen was afraid that if she had taken them to task and the discussion resulted in firing or resignation, she'd have no one to fulfill their duties. As a result, their behavior had gone unchallenged.

So rather than address the matter head-on with Starr and her coworker, Helen had written me to evaluate Dan's (and my) perception of the situation. And when I reported that Dan couldn't explain his anger in Pizza King and told me that he wanted to drop the issue and expressed his willingness to continue to go on outings with Starr, Helen didn't pursue the matter further.

I was livid. This mistreatment of my brother was inexpressibly painful, as was the betrayal of our trust. And the cruelty! I couldn't fathom why someone who had been hired to help people like Dan reclaim a foothold in the broader community would mock him for not having it. Starr and her coworker were being paid to help him participate in the kinds of ordinary activities, like going out for pizza, that had been mostly denied him for much of his life. But instead they had publicly humiliated him so egregiously that those within hearing distance were upset on his behalf. Dan had faced difficulties over the previous forty-one years that these girls couldn't begin to imagine, and their response to him was to twist the knife. That viciousness defied my comprehension.

Much later, I wondered: *had* Dan in fact unintentionally grazed Starr in a way she found disturbing the day before the Pizza King outing? Did she consider her cruelty to him the following day a matter of payback? If so, her assaults on his dignity might have been more intelligible—but still no more justified. Ella had handled Dan's transgressive behavior correctly; she had reported it and refused to work with him again. If Starr believed that Dan had meant to fondle her, she too could have reported it and discontinued contact with him. Instead, she accepted the responsibility of caring for him and then used that opportunity to dehumanize him. I had already guessed that Starr was immature for her age; I just had never imagined that her immaturity would take a sadistic turn.

Dan is brain injured, I thought, and he would never intentionally hurt anyone. (His IED can be hurtful, but those episodes aren't intentional.) Who, then—Dan or Starr—was truly more damaged? Did Starr warrant a measure of compassion, in the wake of whatever outrages slashed and scarred her humanity, leaving her with so little fellow feeling?

But these thoughts came later. At the time of Ella's revelations, I was simply furious—at Starr for her mistreatment of my brother and at Helen for allowing it to go unaddressed, failing both to hold Starr accountable and to inform me of what had happened.

On the phone with me, but without my prompting, Ella expressed an opinion that dovetailed with my own impressions: from the beginning, Starr's conduct toward Dan had been inappropriate. Her demeanor, dress, and physical as well as verbal flirtations had been provocative. As I had expressed it in my journal, Starr had been "teasing him" and "indiscriminately playing with her sexual power," and she needed "to learn how, when, and with whom to exercise it." Still, Dan hadn't been moved to respond to her sexual teasing, because he thought the teasing itself was foolish, haughty, and patronizing.

As soon as Ella and I finished our conversation, I called Carrie, Dan's OBRA service coordinator, telling her about the Pizza King incident. She began filing an incident report while we were still on the phone, and Starr was barred on the spot from having any further contact with Dan—exactly what Helen should have done, I thought.

Within a week, Dan and I met with Carrie and the head of Help at Home, another local OBRA services provider. As we walked together toward the conference room to discuss switching providers, I told Carrie about Dan's inappropriate behavior toward Ella. From the day we met, Carrie had liked Dan and had energetically championed his interests, doing whatever she could to boost his quality of life. I had dreaded telling her about Dan's grab at Ella, worried that he would plummet in Carrie's estimation and that his trespass might bring some sort of sanctions against him. But failing to acknowledge hard realities would have made us less effective partners, and hiding a difficult truth would have been both counterproductive and disrespectful, as it is in all relationships.

But when I confessed Dan's transgression, Carrie didn't even blink. "That kind of behavior is common with TBI," she said. "It's a matter of reduced impulse control. People who work closely with this population have to expect this issue to arise from time to time and be prepared to deal with it in ways that don't compromise the well-being of either party. It's a matter of adequate training." And that was the end of the discussion.

(As a relevant aside, a few weeks earlier, while I was visiting Dan in Harbor's dining hall, an elderly woman at his table beckoned me closer. When I went to her side and leaned down to ask how I could help her, she firmly grasped my bottom and gave it a squeeze, remarking how nice it was. I was not the least bit offended, recognizing that grab for what it was: an unconsidered, unself-conscious attempt to connect. Her lapse in social observance was not a claim of entitlement or an exertion of dominance—not the kind of abuse of social power through sexual trespass that rightly fueled the #MeToo movement. The woman's behavior was inappropriate, certainly, but it didn't qualify as intentional. It was, rather, a neurological lapse of judgment. And I'm confident that, in the years before her cognitive wiring had fallen into disarray, she herself would have been astonished and more than a little dismayed by her own behavior.)

As I learned in the meeting with Carrie and Help at Home, arranging for the provision of reliable OBRA services was more complicated than I had realized. Staffing—in terms of both quantity and quality—is a continual concern for these agencies, because the job is demanding and the salary is low, making it difficult to attract and keep workers who have the ability to secure easier or better-paying employment. (I believe that such work is a heartfelt calling for a rarified few, who find it rewarding in ways that money alone isn't.) As a result of these conditions, turnover is frequent, and oversight can be less than rigorous, with questionable or even bad behavior tolerated because the only possible alternative is to cut clientele. Mid-meeting, I better comprehended the predicament Helen had faced. While I still strongly felt that her decision to disregard Starr's bullying was the wrong choice to make, I at least understood why she had made it.

At the meeting with Carrie and Help at Home, Dan officially terminated his alliance with Indiana Friends and contracted with the new agency, but in succeeding weeks, its program director was unable to secure adequate staffing for Dan's outings. We subsequently met and signed with a third company, Hillcroft. The assistant assigned to Dan was conscientious and kind and got along well with him, but staff availability continued to be a problem and, as a result, Dan's excursions were often canceled. We considered, in fact, a return to Indiana Friends (Starr had been dismissed), but it remained understaffed and so wouldn't have been able to add Dan to its client list even if we had requested it. So Dan remained with Hillcroft, simply enduring the cancellations.

I remain infinitely grateful to OBRA and to the agencies charged with providing services to people who need them, like Dan. The outings infused his life with rediscovered passion, along with the ordinary pleasures most of us take for granted, including regular social interaction. Unfortunately, support agencies with sufficient staffing by compassionate, properly trained personnel seem to be the exception rather than the rule, and we have yet to find that exception. The program directors and managers of the agencies are not to blame; rather, our institutional system is at fault, as it fails to adequately compensate people entrusted with the hands-on care of those whose well-being depends upon public funding. Until wages are commensurate with demands, adequate training is funded, and a career in the industry carries a proper measure of social respect, securing safe and reliable services likely will remain an ongoing challenge. And now I know to be a little less sanguine, a little more cautious, about my faith in those who provide these crucial services. Most of these workers, I believe, while perhaps not driven primarily by compassion, are relatively kind. But some are not. The nature of the field opens gaps that unskilled, unfeeling, unscrupulous people slip into unchecked. It's an imperfect system that, as I have learned, requires oversight and skepticism.

Nevertheless, I'm very grateful it exists.

★ ★ ★

In November, Dan and I made an appointment with Harbor's social worker, who also served as the facility's counselor. I was hoping to get some professional assistance in helping Dan apply CBT strategies to his problem with IED. Because all the literature I found promotes a degree of reading and written homework as critical therapeutic tools, and because Dan can neither read nor write, I wondered if there might be alternative activities that he and I might tackle together that would supply him with similar—or at least some—benefits.

The counselor listened with evident interest as I explained Dan's IED issues, expressed my hope that they might be addressed through CBT, and acknowledged that I don't know enough about counseling tactics to improvise alternatives that would compensate for Dan's inability to read and write. She shook her head sadly and said that she wished she could help, but she had no ideas to offer. I had hoped that even if she had no ready answers, she might explore some of her professional resources—professional literature reporting current research and the latest practices, and maybe colleagues she could discuss Dan's case with—but she didn't seem to consider these possibilities.

"You're a kind woman," she said to me, as she left. Then she turned to Dan and said, "Good luck."

★ ★ ★

Also in November, I gradually became aware that Dan's energy seemed to be waning. He still made his daily walks through Harbor's hallways, ate in the dining hall, and participated in events that appealed to him, but he frequently seemed tired and increasingly listless. I wondered at first if the problem was a mounting depression, as a result of getting out less often following the Indiana Friends debacle. I managed to get him to Agape once before the organization's winter break, but I wouldn't risk a second try. Transferring him and getting the wheelchair into and out of my car on my own had been difficult, stressful, and risky; when we returned to Harbor, I had to leave him clinging to my car's doorframe, hanging halfway in and halfway out of the car, while I bolted inside to get help. I didn't dare repeat the experience, even though Dan angrily insisted we could manage. Dyke and I tried to pick up some of the slack. We often took him out for early dinners on Saturdays, but Dan was now spending nearly all of his time indoors at Harbor—a considerable change from the active schedule that had so revitalized him over the previous months. And he acutely missed riding at Agape.

Still, Dan didn't seem depressed—his sense of humor remained intact, he still enjoyed our visits and dinner outings, and he still pulled his own weight in conversations. He just seemed unusually fatigued. I mentioned my concerns to Dave, who wondered if Dan was simply wearing down. Along with the multiple impairments caused by serious TBI, he noted, survivors are subject to a shortened lifespan. Maybe years of exerting his body to its limits (and often beyond) had prematurely pushed Dan into the last phase of his life. It was wonderful, Dave said, that Dan had been able to experience the life he'd been having in Indiana; his reconnection to horses and his greater engagement in human community had been unmitigated blessings—well worth the relocation. But it might have constituted his last hurrah.

I was crushed at the thought. Was Dan at high risk of early death because of his TBI? Researching the question taught me that longevity for people with moderate to severe TBI is indeed statistically shorter. According to one study, people who sustained their TBI between the ages of fifteen and nineteen, like Dan, faced an overall reduction in life expectancy by nine to eleven years.[1] Many of the problems associated with reduced life expectancy for TBI survivors also afflict people without brain injury; issues that frequently attend TBI also beset the many people with unhealthy lifestyle-related habits such as chronic inactivity, improper nutrition (i.e., obesity or nutritional deficiencies), and the abuse of alcohol or drugs. Also, the compromised executive functioning and poor judgment that many TBI survivors exhibit are not exclusive to brain-injured people, but they can result in unwise choices that lead, sometimes circuitously, to fatal injury. Various physical impairments, by their very nature, such as balance issues or muscle weakness, can increase the chances of lethal accidents, and seizures are also associated with premature mortality in this population. According to the CDC, people with brain injuries are fifty times more likely to die of seizures than other people, eleven times more likely to die of accidental drug poisoning, nine times more likely to die of infections, and six times more likely to die of pneumonia.[2]

So the literature indicates that Dan is in fact at greater risk than the general population of premature mortality, but he is less at risk than many other TBI survivors. Despite the sedentariness imposed by his paralysis and use of a wheelchair, he makes a point of exercising by pushing himself in his wheelchair for several hours every day, building up his muscles, including his heart. He avoids sweets and overeating; his dietary self-control would shame the vast majority of Americans. And while he eats cheeseburgers or pizza on a weekly basis, the rest of his meals consist almost entirely of meat, vegetables, and fruit—again, more nutritionally balanced than is true for the general US population.

But even if Dan followed the reported pattern of a nine-year reduction in lifespan for TBI survivors, he was still statistically young. The average life expectancy for a white American male is seventy-nine years old, twenty years older than Dan. Of course, statistical averages have little correlation with any given individual outcome, so Dan's age at his death can no more be predicted than mine; the statistics reflect mere generalizations, and their predictive value is severely limited—or, to be more precise, immaterial to any individual case.

So my research wasn't especially helpful in getting a sense of what may or may not have been going on with Dan. Was he, after a life full of confronting challenges that often required great physical struggle, simply worn out and winding down? I found no information that addressed that possibility, that made such a hypothesis seem either likely or unlikely. I determined that I would simply stay alert and keep watch.

★ ★ ★

In October, Shiloh resigned as Harbor's administrative director. As I told her later, when I heard she was no longer at Harbor, I felt like a kid coming home from school to learn that her mom had left town without leaving a forwarding address. Shiloh had been the guiding spirit of Harbor, the person who orchestrated the conditions that had made Dan's new residence a home. As Dyke observed early on, Harbor hadn't been just a job for her, but a mission. Her caring engagement and pride in the place had given me confidence. I trusted her sensibilities and valued her oversight. What's more, because of her experience with her own brain-injured mother, she had an uncommon understanding of Dan's problems and was genuinely empathetic, personally interested in his well-being in a way that I doubted any successor would be. And she was unusually open to feedback, always willing to listen to and address any—*any*—issues. I worried that the quality of my brother's experience at Harbor would drop without her there, but the few people I discussed that concern with, including Shiloh herself, assured me that, because I was so involved in his day-to-day life, it was unlikely that much would change for Dan.

There were changes, though. Over the first few months, there was a near exodus of personnel, many of whom had worked at Harbor for years. At the time of Shiloh's departure, I recognized almost all of the people who worked there, knew most of them by name, and shared easy relationships with many. But soon after Shiloh left, the number of faces I didn't recognize began outnumbering those I did. Understaffing had been a perpetual concern, even when Shiloh was in charge (as it is for most, if not all, long-term care facilities). But the nurses and CNAs on Shiloh's watch were overwhelmingly kind, well-trained, diligent, and watchful. Those who weren't didn't stay long. But under the oversight of an interim director, suddenly there was a new, rapidly rotating crop of caregivers, surrounding Dan with people he didn't know and—at least as problematic—who didn't know him. Many of the care providers who had welcomed him to Harbor and helped him to acclimate and feel at home, who had personally contributed to and felt invested in his well-being—they suddenly vanished, replaced by strangers. And while some of the new hires seemed well-trained, attentive, hard-working, and amiable, others were less so. The staffing shortage intensified, but even so, the performance of some of the new staff wouldn't have been tolerated by Shiloh.

I was unsettled by the changes in staff, and not only on Dan's behalf. For me, too, there had been personal as well as pragmatic advantages to being part of the Harbor community. I'd developed friendly relationships with many of the caregivers and other personnel who were now gone, and I missed my sense of community. I discovered that Harbor was not only the place that was helping my brother to thrive but it had been helping me thrive too, as an integral part of my own social world. But now I was presented with a stream of new names and faces to learn, without knowing who would be returning the following week and who wouldn't. I was now a stranger to most of those I approached with Dan's concerns. Instead of feeling like a team member with shared goals, I suspected I often was viewed as just another family member with a penchant for complaining.

Fortunately, the turbulence began to wane after several months. The churn of new names and faces slowed a bit. A few of the new staff members took a real interest in Dan, liked him, and viewed him (and me) as someone they were glad to work with. Whenever possible, I still tended to seek out the old guard, relying on them for information and assistance, but as the weeks passed there were fewer and fewer of that contingent. Still, over time, the new climate began to feel more familiar, and my confidence in the new administrators and Dan's new caregivers began, if slowly, to build. But in Shiloh's wake, my sense that Dan (and I) had found the perfect niche at Harbor waned.

★ ★ ★

Toward the end of November, Dan, Dyke, and I received invitations to Agape's annual Christmas party for the organization's staff and clientele, along with their families. Harbor informed us that, because the activity director was on medical leave, there would be no Christmas party for residents this year, so other than going to church with Dyke and me on Christmas Eve and a small family Christmas Day get-together at a local restaurant, Agape's party would be Dan's only holiday event.

Many Harbor residents (or their families) had hung Christmas wreaths or other festive baubles on their doors both to personalize their space and to mark the holiday season. Dan never cared about decorating his door, so his plastic over-the-door hanger still bore the Panama hat that activities staff had suspended there in mid-April, to commemorate Kentucky Derby Day. For some reason, seven months later the hat suddenly snagged my attention. "That hat doesn't express you very well," I said. "Wouldn't you rather have a cowboy hat hanging on that hook?"

At first Dan merely shrugged at the suggestion, but a few moments later he nodded. It wasn't a pressing concern, we agreed, but if there was going to be a hat hanging on his door, a cowboy hat was more appropriate. Suddenly inspired, I noted that, if we got the hat now, he could also wear it to Agape's Christmas party. He liked the idea.

I sat on his bed and opened a browser on my iPhone. Still thinking mostly in terms of a door decoration, I scanned Halloween Cowboy-costume accessories. But by this time, Dan had something else in mind: if he were going to wear the hat to the Christmas party, he wanted a nice one.

One idea led to another, and before the afternoon was out, we had ordered a Bailey Premium Wool Felt cowboy hat in chocolate brown, a cowboy-cut Wrangler shirt in finely woven indigo denim with pearl snaps, and a two-toned silver belt buckle etched with a racing horse in mid-gallop, his rider in full crouch over the saddle.

All through the next week, I impatiently tracked packages and kept watch for shipments, eager to deliver the elements of Dan's new outfit. Every item arrived on time and as advertised. When I showed Dan his new hat, he was pleased, but he spelled "STEAM." I learned that new cowboy hats are sold with flat brims, so that their wearers can customize them to suit their personal preferences, which required shaping the hat over clouds of steam. Dan wanted his brim curved upward on the sides. I was hesitant; I knew nothing about the process and was afraid I might ruin his expensive new hat, but he assured me that shaping hats was "EASY." And a DIY website explicitly assured me that I couldn't fail badly enough to destroy the hat. Nor did I. After fifteen minutes with a hot teakettle, a pair of dishwashing gloves, and a pounding heart, I was happy with the results. And Dan seemed pleased enough.

December 13 finally arrived. When Dyke and I got to Dan's room to pick him up, he was downright dashing in midnight-blue jeans and matching new shirt. But we encountered a momentary snag: a few weeks earlier, I had measured Dan's belt to make sure it still fit, but I must have erred; the belt, which he hadn't worn in decades, was too small by inches to buckle. On the spot, Dyke took off his belt and we snapped in Dan's new silver buckle. It fit Dan perfectly and looked great. He put on the hat, its brim nattily upturned, and we were ready to go.

The hour-long drive in the car felt less convivial than I had expected. I chattered away, but Dan's energy level that evening was decidedly low. When I asked if he were feeling okay, he answered, "SORE." Although Dan usually found Dyke's car roomy and comfortable, maybe the long ride, I thought, was at fault. I hoped that he would feel more comfortable once we arrived at Agape and he was back in his wheelchair. Throughout the trip, we listened to country music on the radio, and I kept up the small talk, but I was anxious for the drive to end—and Dan was unmistakably more so.

When we arrived at Agape, the crowd was substantial, and parking was scarce. We were heartily greeted at the door; all evening, Agape staff and volunteers fussed over Dan as though he were a rock star, and he received their attentions with pleased humility. The riding arena and barn were bedecked with fragrant pine sprigs and wreaths, shiny ornaments, calico bows, and scattered straw. We were directed first to the stalls, where Dan and Bo nuzzled companionably for a few minutes, establishing a momentary bubble of quiet amid the din and bustle, each seeming calmed by the other. Then we pushed into the riding arena and settled down at a table. As we ate—Dan had a scant cup of chili and two chocolate chip cookies, one of which he wrapped in a napkin for later—Agape personnel entertained the crowd with a campy Western-themed performance of the "Twelve Days of Christmas." Afterward, a number of people acquainted with Dan dropped by our table to chat and introduce their spouses and children. The community was open-hearted and accepting, and it embraced Dyke and me because it so warmly embraced Dan.

Throughout the evening, though, Dan was unusually low-key. I watched him with growing concern, as he became increasingly fatigued, to the point that I wondered several times if he had fallen asleep. At one point I feared that perhaps he had passed out, but he answered when I vigorously shook his arm. Still, he was affable when visitors dropped by our table, and when Dyke asked him if he'd like to grab a Five Guys cheeseburger on the way home since he'd eaten so little at the party, he brightened. I wondered then if he were simply tired and hungry.

By the time we got back to Harbor with his burger, it was nine-thirty. Dan finished eating about an hour later and was thoroughly exhausted, longing for bed. This time, I was happy to help him; he was so fatigued that waiting twenty minutes or so for a CNA was simply out of the question. Dyke and I undressed him, set him up with his toothbrush and related gear, and said our good nights. Agape's party hadn't been the high point for him that I had hoped it would be, but I was glad we went. I was also, by this time, glad the evening was over.

Just after the Christmas party, at my request, Dan was examined by Harbor's doctor and he received an extensive panel of blood tests. The results suggested that, in terms of blood chemistry, he was in excellent health, with a profile that most fifty-nine-year-olds would envy. Yet he still languished.

As it turned out, Dan's listlessness and aches had been caused by a series of viruses. They walloped him, lingering for five or six weeks before he gradually regained his strength and customary vitality. But it was a bad season for the flu in Muncie. Dan, Dyke, and I had all received flu shots in October, but we all succumbed to the circulating strain. I was the only one of us tested, but the results were positive. While Dyke, fortunately, snapped back to health after a few days, recovery for both Dan and me was slower. At length, Dan's energy and enthusiasm returned. And by the time Agape's winter break was over in early January, Dan was hotly anticipating his rides with Bo.

Notes

1. Cynthia Harrison-Felix, et al., "Life Expectancy Following Rehabilitation" *Journal of Head Trauma Rehabilitation* 27, no. 6 (November 2012). doi: 10.1097/htr.0b013e3182738010
2. "Moderate to Severe Traumatic Brain Injury Is a Lifelong Condition" *Centers for Disease Control and Prevention*. www.cdc.gov/traumaticbraininjury/pdf/moderate_to_severe_tbi_lifelong-a.pdf

10 The Power of Belongingness

The photos tell a story:

June 1978: Five months before his accident, Dan is in bed, propped against pillows, bedspread pulled up to his chin. His tanned forearms are just visible among the covers, and he holds a paperback in his hands. His face slightly swiveled away from the book he's reading, he steadily eyes the photographer (most likely Dad) as if to say, Something I can help you with? Both his eyes and his hair are the color of dark chocolate, and thick, wavy curls tumble just over the tops of his ears. He looks younger than his eighteen years. A whisper of a mustache hovers over his lips, which are full and red, a tolerant, slight smile lurking just under their surface.

May 1979: Six months after his injury, in St. Jude's Hospital in Fullerton, California, Dan stands between Mom on his left and me on his right, his arms curved around our necks for support. I'm in profile with one of my hands slipped around his back, the other positioned lightly over the hand he has draped over my shoulder. Mom grasps his waist with one hand, the other splayed over his ribcage, holding him firmly in place. He will not fall. A white band around his neck supports the plastic tracheotomy tube in his throat just above the v-neck of his t-shirt, which is darkened by a thin stream of saliva flowing from his mouth. Although neither Mom nor I realize it at the time, his gold basketball shorts are wet at the crotch. His hair is mussed, covering the large pink scar on his scalp. Both Mom and I are looking up at his face, our own faces seeking the means to smile but not finding it. Dan is the only one looking at the camera. The smile he offers is skewed by the effort it's taking him to stay on his feet.

June 1979: A few weeks later, still at St. Jude's, Dan's having a better day. This close-up shows Dan from the waist up, sitting on a salmon vinyl couch. He's had a haircut, and a fringe of dark hair falls neatly over his upper forehead. The pink t-shirt he wears bears an illustration of a butterfly on a flower and is captioned "New Life," a gift that exemplifies my

DOI: 10.4324/9781003340294-10

desperate cheerleading in this period, evidence of my frenetic desperation to change the story. Except for the trachea tube and the dampness staining his shirt, he looks no different than he had a year earlier. He gazes steadily into the camera, his expression wide open, eyes serious but lips parted with the ghost of a smile. In this captured moment, there is no hint of all he has lost. He is so beautiful I could weep. And when alone, at the time, I often did.

Fall 1980: Slightly less than a year and a half later, Dan sits outdoors in a vinyl-slatted lounge chair at a camp for people with impairments. Wheelchairs abound. Dan is dressed neatly in jeans and a navy-blue t-shirt. His posture is exemplary. A white towel is draped around his neck, a constant accessory he uses to wipe his mouth every few minutes. It keeps his shirt dry. A jockey helmet with a personalized leather cover sits on his lap, a gift from our parents to protect his head in case he falls, which he seldom does now. But he wisely wears the helmet anyway whenever he walks unassisted or rides his three-wheeled cruising bike. His face is a study in open delight: with a huge grin, he brandishes his cane, appearing to snare in its crook the neck of a middle-aged man seated beside him, who is mugging for the camera. In this moment, at least, there is joy in his life.

December 1980: In the first of a pair of photos, Dan stands balanced in the doorway of his red Toyota truck, arm lifted in a friendly wave, smiling broadly. In this photo too, his posture is perfect. He's in a short-sleeved colorblocked polo and jeans, appropriate for the mildly warm Southern California winters. In the second shot, taken a few minutes later, he's in the driver's seat, arm casually draped across the open window frame. He glows with vitality and health, and a bypasser would see only a good-looking kid, perhaps attributing the towel around his neck to an imminent tennis match. Judging from his smile, he's on his way to somewhere he's glad to be going.

December 1982: Dan stands in front of a Christmas tree. Despite the holiday decorations surrounding him, he gazes solemnly into the camera, back straight, lightly leaning on a cane with his left hand, his right arm enclosed in a cast. Surgeons have cut tendons in his right wrist in hopes of relieving its spasticity. When the cast is removed weeks after this photo is taken, he will discover he has permanently lost all function in this hand. He's in Georgia now and, at least in this photo, has lost much of the sparkle he displayed in his truck two years earlier.

Fall 1987: Just shy of nine years after the accident, Dan is leaning against his truck, now a blue Toyota, in our parents' driveway. Dave, smiling heartily into the camera after buddy-walking with Dan, stands in profile a foot or so from his brother. Dad makes a rare appearance in the background, for once in front of the camera rather than behind it. Hands in his back pockets, he is regarding his sons, not the camera, and stands at the ready to assist if needed. Dan's torso curves forward, neck bent so that his chin hovers just above his chest, head angled slightly toward his right shoulder. His posture is no longer perfect. His useless right hand angles sharply backward toward his elbow. It looks painful, but it isn't, because he has very little feeling on that side of his body. His eyes glance upward, allowing him to cast his effort at a smile toward the camera. He can't quite manage it. Clearly, the preceding few years have been hard on him, and soon Dad will find a buyer for his truck. Dan will keenly mourn the loss.

July 2002: Dan is the ring bearer at Dyke's and my outdoor wedding. It's 103° in the shade of Savannah's moss-draped live oaks. Dan has signed out of the hospital for the afternoon, still recuperating from his fall in the kitchen of his Oliver Place apartment, where he had lived for the previous eleven years. Dave, who escorted me to Dyke's side, will return Dan to the hospital after our reception lunch. None of us, including Dan, knows where he will live when he's released from the hospital. Dan's in a bright white short-sleeved dress shirt, navy-blue dress pants, and a blue and silver striped tie. His hospital identification band is on his wrist. He has insisted on holding our rings as planned. He's wilting in his wheelchair, but he's both determined and glad to take part in this momentous occasion in my life. I'm profoundly touched and grateful.

April 2017: Fast-forward 15 years: in his room at Trinity Village, having recently decided to spend not only his nights but also his days in bed, Dan lies on his back with a pillow wedged under his head. He is unclothed except for a sheet covering him from his belly down, and he is thin, but not yet emaciated. The bend in his neck pulls his head upward off the pillow and angles it severely to the right, his ear almost touching his shoulder. His paralyzed arm rests on his chest, wrist bent backward and hand clenched shut. He is unshaven, as he relies on others for his shaves, but his close-cropped hair is neatly brushed, as he can do that himself. Eyes nearly closed, he is laughing broadly toward Dave behind the camera, who has apparently said something Dan finds uproarious. The room is dim, with faint afternoon light struggling to make its way through slatted window blinds. The concrete block walls behind him are a muddy ochre. Dan looks like a critically ill patient in a hospital bed caught in one of his last gasps of levity, but he's in the room he's called home for eleven years.

February 2018: Dan is in bed again, this time clothed in a mint-green hospital gown. His head is still raised from the pillow and bent toward his right shoulder, right arm still angled across his chest, wrist still arched backward and hand still clenched into a tight fist. His hair is uncharacteristically long, with dark curls highlighted by slivers of silver. My forearm appears in the frame of the photo, offering him a glass of milk, and his gaunt left wrist is bent to accept it. He is laughing toward Dyke behind the camera. Sunlight floods the bed, almost as bright as Dan's mood. He's finishing his first breakfast at Harbor Health, and there's no mistaking his delight.

Following Dan's arrival in Indiana, Dyke and I took many photos on my phone, largely to share with Dave. There are photos of Dan's room, painted in warm, saturated tones and adorned with photos and treasured artifacts from his life: the monogrammed jockey helmet our parents gave him decades ago; the winning ticket he bought betting on a horse that he co-owned with Will Swift, the trainer he was working for when he sustained his injury; the small bronze statue of a jockey riding a horse in full gallop; a world globe that Dyke and I gave him for Christmas years ago; a horseshoe someone at Harbor has given him. Dan decided the arrangement of these objects, telling me where to place each piece, adjusting their positioning by fractions of an inch until he was aesthetically satisfied.

A few other photos from Indiana:

March 2018: Three weeks after his arrival at Harbor, Dan is sitting in a chair, clean and clean-shaven, hair closely shorn on the sides and just a bit longer on top, dressed in jeans and a faded red t-shirt. Eleven months earlier at Trinity Village, he had decided that the pain and effort of getting out of bed and putting on clothes weren't worth whatever modest pleasure and considerable soreness sitting up entailed. But the smile he offers Dave, who will momentarily receive the digital photo, is as bright as the room he sits in. He looks some twenty-five years younger than his fifty-eight years, and he's demonstrating why certain smiles are characterized as "radiant."

April 2018: Dan is in bed on his nightly call with Dave, phone pressed to his ear, laughing wholeheartedly at something his brother has just said. Dan's face lights up every time Dave calls. I don't know that Dan would have survived the years preceding his relocation to Harbor without Dave's enduring presence in his life. Dan is indisputably tough, but he's still human, with the human need for intimate connection and belongingness. His relationship with Dave sustained his spirit through years of rejection and isolation. The bond between them, already ironclad in earliest childhood, had deepened and solidified over years when Dave was closer to Dan than anyone else in his life. That bond continues to be a central mainstay for them both—unshakable and irreplaceable. And Dave's calls continue to bring Dan the kind of elation that bubbles through this photo.

May 2018: It's Farm Day at Harbor Health, and Dan is in the parking lot on a warm and sunny spring evening. *Photo 1:* Cimarron the horse nuzzles Dan's hand; his other hand touches the horse's shoulder with the gentle assurance of a horseman. Dan is in quarter profile, obscuring most of his face, and although his right hand and arm are still clutched across his chest, his head is mostly upright now, no longer listing so severely toward his shoulder, and it thrusts a bit less sharply forward. *Photo 2:* Still at Farm Day, Dan is laughing broadly as TC, another horse, licks the top of his head. Dan's delight is palpable, even through the entirely visual medium of a digital camera. Those around him (including me) are laughing with him, enjoying his interaction with TC almost as much as Dan himself. But not quite.

May 2018: A week later Dan, in his wheelchair, is strapped securely in the back of a transport van on our way back to Harbor. He's just completed his first visit to a dentist in over a decade. The dental technician meticulously cleaned his teeth, and the dentist complimented him on the condition of his mouth, especially considering the long lapse in his dental care. On this return trip to Harbor, I've told him I want to capture his "pearly whites" on camera for Dave. Mouth wide open, lips pulled back to expose as many teeth as possible, eyes scrunched closed in the effort, he is mugging, belly-laughing.

There are many more photos. As the months pass, Dan is increasingly less gaunt as he puts on thirty-five sorely needed pounds, arriving at the point where he closely monitors his diet so he doesn't gain more. One of my favorite photos is a three-person selfie close-up taken in January 2019, a month shy of the first anniversary of Dan's arrival in Indiana. Dan looms large in the foreground, with my face thrust over his shoulder and Dyke's face over my shoulder, all three of us wide-eyed and gaping, clowning for the camera. It's a moment of thorough exuberance, a moment in which all three of us glow with the joyous well-being that accompanies a constant, secure sense of delight in each other, in our mutual belonging.

★ ★ ★

These photos don't, of course, tell the full story. No snapshot ever does. Life isn't a fairy tale, and Dan still has problems—serious problems—arising from his TBI. He deals with a number of primary impairments that stem from the neurological fallout of brain injury itself. Hemiplegia complicates the most mundane activities of his daily life even as it entirely rules out others, preventing him from participating in many of the pastimes he once enjoyed. Dysarthria, dysphagia, and his modest reduction in cognitive processing speed lead others to misjudge his levels of awareness, intelligence, and relational competence. He's unable to correct such misperceptions because, along with dysarthria, aphasia prevents him from speaking. Anosognosia, both a curse and a blessing, causes him to reject certain adaptive tools and other kinds of assistance and advice that would alleviate some of his hardships, but it also motivates him to accomplish goals that signify real, measurable progress, and it provides a foothold for his characteristic optimism. Finally, IED explosions continually threaten to compromise his relationships with the caregivers who must deal with the fallout. And although his outbursts never really jeopardize the relationships within our family, they do at times cause quickly passing but decidedly unpleasant emotional distress.

Dan also deals with secondary issues that arise from these primary impairments. His hemiplegia forces sedentariness, which increases his risk of developing heart disease, obesity, cancer, Type 2 diabetes, and osteoporosis. (To his great credit, though, he works hard to forestall these effects through dietary self-control and exercise, spending hours each day propelling himself in his wheelchair.) In addition, continual sitting can cause or exacerbate insomnia, urinary incontinence, and pressure sores that often cause him considerable pain. Aphasia and dysarthria make it difficult, and sometimes impossible, for him to discuss problems as they arise to obtain specific kinds of help. They also preclude most reading—not only reading for pleasure but also reading that gives him access to health and safety information he might find useful. Dysphagia increases his chances of choking when he eats or drinks.

In addition to these primary and secondary conditions, all of these impairments have grave social consequences in that they undermine Dan's self-presentation—the impression of him that is grasped and evaluated by others. The negative reactions of others thwart his efforts to shape a healthy identity and compromise his social standing. As a result of his neurological injuries, Dan has been repeatedly infantilized, excluded, rejected, neglected, and even bullied. And, doubtlessly, these social reactions have caused him at least as much distress as any of the physical impairments he faces—in fact, as he has indicated, considerably more.

★ ★ ★

Although it's not evident to people who don't know him, in most respects Dan is thoroughly "normal." (This is true especially considering the well-justified point made by disability studies scholars that the characteristics we use to assign normality exist on a continuum. Accidents, diseases, and the effects of aging cause some degree of impairment at various times in nearly everyone's life. Consequently, impairment itself is normal, at least sometimes, for almost all of us.) Dan is normal in the ways that are of chief importance to us all: he has always and ever had the same kinds of needs, desires, and dreams that typify human existence. Since his injury, though, he's had a much harder time gratifying his needs, satisfying his desires, and fulfilling his dreams, because most of our needs, desires, and dreams hinge on social integration and interpersonal relationships.

It's worth a brief aside here to note that disability scholars and rights advocates differentiate between the states of *having impairments* and of *being disabled*. An *impairment* is an immutable characteristic that prevents a person from engaging in some activity that most people take for granted, like walking or speaking. *Disability*, on the other hand, is the endurance of (1) the societal failure to construct or adjust environments to make it easier for people with impairments to more fully participate in their society and (2) the acculturated attitude that causes social members to withhold the baseline regard that we typically offer our other fellow members, from people with impairments. In other words, impairment is imposed by an accident, disease, congenital anomaly, or other physiological, neurological, psychological, or cognitive condition; disability is a status imposed by other members of society who view (and consequently treat) people with impairments as lesser human beings.

Responses others have to Dan sometimes take the form of pity. Social psychologists and other scholars distinguish pity from empathy. Empathy is, in effect, sharing someone's experience of hardship *with* them, bringing the empathizer into the same psychosocial space as that person, eliminating the emotional distance between them. Pity, on the other hand, is feeling sorry *for* someone—acknowledging a person's hardship but maintaining a psychic distance by staying *above* (or at least outside) the person's experience, rather than understanding them through sharing in their feelings. In his description of the defining characteristics of pity, philosophy and medical bioethics professor Robert Kimball writes, "[P]ity includes an element of psychological distancing . . . and may include an element of revulsion, superiority, or even contempt."[1] There is an element of "There but for the grace of God go I"—an attitude that may disguise itself as empathy even as it (unwittingly) distinguishes the speaker as a recipient of God's grace, and the speaker's target as one who is bereft of it, and so apparently not deserving it. Most people on the receiving end of pity know what that pity reflects, even if those reflecting it do not.

While empathy toward TBI survivors is a more appropriate (and the best) response, pity is less damaging than some of the other reactions they are sometimes subjected to. Social psychologists make a distinction among some of those reactions: *ostracism, social exclusion, rejection,* and *bullying*.[2] The public at large tends to use these words interchangeably, but they are distinct reactions with overlapping but distinct consequences, and they all diminish their target's sense of belonging.

The utter disregard called *ostracism* is behavior that ignores someone—that willfully overlooks their presence, signaling that they aren't worth acknowledging. This reaction is the polar opposite of empathy. Ostracism sends the message that, in effect, that person doesn't merit even the minimal interaction that we extend to strangers who, simply because they are our fellow human beings, merit a claim to our attention (e.g., to ask for directions or to receive an apology if they are bumped into). *Social exclusion* doesn't refuse attention, but it does deny the kinds of accepting interaction expected by those included within a social circle. The presence of those who are excluded may be acknowledged, but the acknowledgment they receive is perfunctory or grudging. *Rejection* is conduct that lets targets know that they are deemed somehow unacceptable for involvement in a relationship or for belonging within a social network. And finally, *bullying* refers to overtly abusive actions inflicted with the intention to harm a person, whether the aggression is verbal, nonverbal, or physical (or all three).

I could cite specific instances in which Dan has been the object of pity, ostracism, exclusion, rejection, and bullying, and I'm sure he could cite geometrically more. But many, if not most, people—despite their good intentions—interact with Dan as though he were a "BABY," a style of interaction called *infantilization*. Dan is, and views himself as, an adult man, and what's more, a man who has lived forty-three of his sixty-one years facing down a continual onslaught of seemingly intolerable challenges with a degree of courage and persistence that would do any of us credit. To treat Dan like a child fails to respect or even recognize the experience he has accrued and the practical wisdom he has consequently gained over the course of his lifetime. Disability rights advocate Creigh Farinas, whose sister Caley is autistic, has compiled a list of the "top six" responses that characterize the social act of infantilization, which she describes as behavior toward adults with impairments that is "inherently related to not taking someone seriously."[3] Repeatedly, I have seen Dan receive all six of these reactions over the years, some more frequently than others. Quoting Farinas, these forms of interaction infantilize:

1. "Talking to someone like they're a child (or worse yet, a pet)";
2. "Over-simplifying vocabulary or over-explaining concepts";
3. "Denying the person the right to have adult speech patterns, habits, or desires";
4. "Addressing another adult or caregiver instead of the impaired adult themselves";
5. "Not taking a person's opinions, beliefs, or desires seriously"; [and]
6. "Not allowing them to be independent."

Although infantilization is typically an unintentional behavior stemming from an unconsidered and likely subconscious attitude, it nevertheless operates as a form of social exclusion or rejection, in that its target is unmistakably deemed as insufficiently capable of adult interactions because of their impairments. Not surprisingly, when Dan is infantilized, he may respond with an IED outburst, because these forms of interaction are signs of underestimation, lack of respect, and denial of dignity. And yet he has learned to tolerate a degree of infantilization, even though he's aware of the implicit insult to his competence and the unwitting sense of superiority that generates it. He recognizes that those who talk down to him (behaviors #1 and #2 on Farinas's list) typically mean well, unlike those who treat him with the contempt of ostracism, exclusion, rejection, or bullying. Still, the person who infantilizes, however unintentionally, by definition downgrades their interactant's status and undermines their identity.

I know first-hand that those who perpetrate this strain of infantilization may mean well. In January of 2003, when I spent a week of days with Dan at Taylor Heights, the first nursing home he lived in, I was deeply dismayed to realize in retrospect that I had committed this offense against a Taylor Heights resident. In my 2003 master's thesis, I recounted the episode:

> In the hallway on my way to lunch, I pass by the cafeteria. At the doorway, a woman in a faded red fleece sweatsuit signals to me from her wheelchair: with one hand, she frantically grabs at the air in my direction; her eyes are wide and desperate, and her mouth opens and closes soundlessly. I stop, lean toward her, take her hand. "What's the matter, baby? You want to go into the cafeteria?" I ask, and the words and the tone of my voice, as though I were addressing a toddler, sound wrong in my own ears. But she just nods anxiously, eyes still panicky, mouth still working fruitlessly. . . .
>
> Later, at lunch, my own response to her—"What's the matter, baby? You want to go into the cafeteria?"—horrifies me with its condescension. If this woman is lucid—if she is simply aphasic, like my brother—it must appall her to be spoken to like that. With a few thoughtless words, I have mirrored her shift in status: from respected elder, perhaps family matriarch or retired businesswoman, teacher, or community leader, to incoherent supplicant. I addressed her as though she were pre-verbal, infantile, and utterly incompetent, rather than—as is certainly possible—as a sensible elderly woman with a speech disorder. Encountering her within the context of the nursing home, I had assumed the worst. And if I did misjudge her, her

inability to speak prevented her from correcting me, from defending her assailed integrity.

Over lunch, I consider the power we all have to help or hinder each other's self-construction, and I recognize, to my shame, that I have just abused that power.

Without question, I wanted to help. I meant well. But my unthinking response to that woman was infantilization (a concept I wouldn't learn about until years later but nevertheless recognized at the time as feeling "wrong"). I responded to her inability to speak, to competently use language (an inability which we associate with pre-verbal infants and toddlers), and her physical helplessness as I would to a child in distress. I suppose my reaction was "natural" enough, but it was demeaning. At least I learned from this lesson.

The coronavirus quarantine of nursing homes in the spring of 2020 brought to a head the issue of people infantilizing Dan. When I was suddenly informed that Harbor Health was on lockdown—no one except staff could enter or exit the building, effectively barring me—I worried about how Dan would tolerate the restrictions. After all, his thrice-weekly outings, especially his horseback riding at Agape, had injected his life with more variety, enjoyment, and vitality than he had experienced in years. And my regular visits, as instrumental as they often were, were more about reveling in our relationship than anything else. I feared that the abrupt discontinuation of these experiences might lead to either depression or a potentially alienating increase in IED outbursts.

When I expressed my concerns on the phone with his nurse Marjorie, she sought to reassure me that Harbor personnel wouldn't allow him to feel isolated. "He's still going up and down the hallways all day long in his wheelchair," she said, "and whenever he passes by, someone tickles his belly and laughs with him."

"About that . . ." I heard myself saying, without really intending to. I had often witnessed this belly-tickling when Dan and I went through the halls together. Dan indeed responded with good-natured smiles and laughter. But when I first experienced this behavior with him, and I asked him privately in his room how he felt about the prodding and poking, he told me that he viewed the behavior as "SILLY." But he knew that those who interacted with him this way meant only to be friendly, so he accepted their overtures in the spirit in which they were intended. When I asked him if he wanted me to discuss this behavior with someone at Harbor Health in an attempt to change it, he thought a moment before answering "NO." True, the pokes and tickles were silly and even demeaning, but he had come to Harbor two years earlier from a place where he had been roundly excluded, rejected, and finally ostracized—drugged and left alone to lie in bed all day, every day (except for the saving grace of Dave's weekly visits), staring at the ceiling, listening to a television he couldn't turn to see, a bystander to his own life, which was receding even as he watched. If infantilization in the form of some well-intentioned tickling was the price of acceptance, however deficient, he didn't consider it too much to pay. The tickling was at least a sign of welcome, an indication that he was considered a valued part of the Harbor community—even if it also signaled that he was not understood and that his competence and the significance of his sixty years of experience were being overlooked rather than respected.

On the day of the coronavirus lockdown, without forethought, I explained to Marjorie that while both Dan and I understood that when people tickled his belly they meant well, it would be more satisfying for Dan if they would interact with him more age-appropriately—and Dan was a full-grown man. (He turned sixty on the second day of the lockdown.) I repeated several times throughout the conversation, as emphatically as I knew how, that both Dan and I knew that this form of connecting with him was coming from a good place—a place of kindness and good intentions—and we truly appreciated the goodwill that engendered it. But, I said, Dan didn't see himself as a child, which the tickling implied. My interactions with him as an equal, I continued, reaffirmed his adult identity, and I was concerned that, because I wouldn't be permitted to visit for the foreseeable future, he might be distressed by a situation in which the only interactions he had were infantilizing (and I did use that word).

At first, Marjorie was surprised—even shocked—but as I continued explaining, she responded well. "I can see that," she said. "I'll pass the word along."

"When you do," I said, "*please* also include that we've known all along that the tickling was meant only to be kind, and that Dan genuinely appreciates the good-heartedness it comes from."

She promised she would, adding, "It's a teachable moment."

"Exactly!" I replied, remembering my own teachable moment at Taylor Heights. It was the perfect frame.

Later that afternoon, I relayed my conversation with Marjorie to Dan. He approved of the effort, but he doubted anything would change. Infantilization had been a part of his life ever since the accident, and he assumed it was one of those unchangeable things he had to accept. "Well, let's hope for the best," I said. "Let's see if there's any difference in the way people greet you on your walks over the next few days."

The next afternoon, I asked if he'd noticed any change, and he answered, "MAYBE."

When the unit manager, Donna, called me that weekend (for an unrelated reason), she too answered my concerns about the effects of the lockdown by mentioning the belly-tickling as a positive behavior that would keep Dan's spirits up. I told her what I'd told Marjorie a few days earlier. Donna, too, was initially surprised but quickly understood, suggesting as Marjorie had that we'd been gifted a teachable moment. I stressed again that we knew this form of greeting came from a friendly, well-meaning place, and we didn't want to embarrass anybody. She said that it was a good lesson to learn.

Several days later, I again asked Dan if he'd noticed any change in the way people were greeting him in the hallways, and he said, "SOME." I asked if they were still friendly and if he liked the change. To both questions he again answered, "YES," and then laughed. It seemed to be working out, and he was glad the point had been made that he's a man, not a toddler (or a pet), and it was a relief for him to be recognized as capable of adult interactions.

At this point, I was only sorry it had taken me twenty-five months to address it.

★ ★ ★

Infantilization diminishes and demeans people, but it arises from a misunderstanding of their capabilities, and at least some forms of it demonstrate goodwill. Ostracism, exclusion, rejection, and bullying, on the other hand, explicitly involve disparagement. Those who are targeted by these behaviors understand their import, which ranges from dismissive dislike to hostile aggression. That understanding itself is hurtful and destructive.

As I noted previously, because human beings are a radically social species, membership within a social group or community is vitally important to us. For millennia, in a very literal sense, belonging within the group has been a matter of survival. Some researchers suggest that the pain of exclusion or rejection from one's peers is experienced in the same way as physical pain, a neurological phenomenon that stems from our evolutionary development.[4] Social pain theorists propose that because group membership is necessary to an individual's well-being, recognition of separation from the group is accompanied by sensory pain. The evolutionary advantage of this pain, the theory goes, is that it motivates the outcast to change whatever is deemed socially offensive in order to secure group acceptance. Social pain, then, has the same function as physical pain: to prompt remedial action to fix an intolerable situation. Just as physical pain spurs action to alleviate it—not walking on a broken foot, for example—pain caused by social exclusion or rejection also spurs remedial action.

The person experiencing social pain is motivated to change whatever character attributes or behavior others find unacceptable, bringing them into the protective social fold. Moreover, while the pain caused by our need to be accepted as part of a community is an evolutionary legacy from our prehistoric ancestors, it still serves the same purpose, and it is just as vividly experienced by contemporary humans.

To summarize the theory, we are wired so that the various forms of social disconnection cause pain severe enough to compel change. We are incentivized to alter ourselves—our demeanor, our behavior, our speech, our appearance—so that we will be accepted by the group or community we aspire to belong to. Only that acceptance will alleviate the pain of refused belonging.

So consider the plight of the person who is strongly motivated but ontologically unable to change in order to fulfill social expectations—someone who is neurologically or physiologically incapable of adjusting in ways that would bring them into the circle of belonging. When change is not an option, there can be no escape from social pain. As social psychologists Kipling Williams, Joseph Forgas, and William von Hippel point out, being on the receiving end of ostracism, exclusion, rejection, or bullying is "among the most devastating experiences a person can endure."[5] Furthermore, the theory suggests that because sustained psychic pain causes *physiological* changes in cognition and self-regulation, and because these changes are maladaptive, it triggers further social exclusion. In effect, that person is caught in a loop: exclusion causes pain, which causes (or exacerbates) neurological changes in thinking and behavior, which intensifies the exclusion, which causes more pain, and so on.

Until, perhaps, that person is fully excluded and chemically restrained, set out of the way to dissolve until nothing is left of them except their loneliness.

★ ★ ★

Dan's experience at Harbor Health demonstrates that even after years of social disconnection, at least sometimes the cycle that perpetuates loneliness can be broken, and wounds can heal. In the case of someone like Dan, whose linguistic, physical, and behavioral impairments make it impossible for him to conform to normative community expectations, that process requires an empathetic understanding of the psychosocial as well as the physical effects of his TBI by those around him. Fostering that understanding, as in Dan's case, may require intervention.

As I see it, the intervention that brought Dan greater belongingness was composed of six essential elements:

First: *Physical removal.* Dan left the toxic environment of a facility where his full humanity went unrecognized, where he was ostracized, excluded, rejected, and bullied by at least some of those he depended upon for his essential care. He had been bedridden for ten months by the time he moved to Harbor, and his hospitalization for sepsis and his diagnosis of malnourishment ten weeks earlier lead me to doubt that he would have survived much longer had he remained at Trinity Village. At some point years before, the aperture through which Dan might have entered into a relation of belonging in that community had closed.

When Dan arrived at Harbor, the emotional as well as physical care that he received revitalized him. In February of 2018, he was a frail and medically fragile 108 pounds; in less than two years, he had become healthy and hardy, watching his weight and exercising for hours every day on his treks through the facility's maze of hallways. He received long-needed physical therapy that enabled him to regain some of the ground he had lost over years, not only improving some aspects of his somatic well-being but also restoring his characteristic optimism and resilience. He felt physically and psychologically better than he had not least of all because he got a fresh start in a community that welcomed him as one of its own.

Second: *Understanding through narrative.* From the night Dan arrived at Harbor, I told his story to everyone who would listen. I related it piecemeal, allowing circumstances to dictate which aspects were relevant to the moment. Character, plot, setting, conflict, resolution: Dan's life inherently lends itself to the telling. I discovered that his story further circulated among personnel at Harbor; in the first few months, staff members I had never met approached me with comments or questions about Dan's life that invited elaboration. Clearly, sharing his experiences with others helped them to identify and empathize with him, which helped to weave him into the social mesh of his new home.

Third: *Understanding through knowledge.* In exploring bodies of research that have developed over recent years in various fields, I learned a lot about TBI and the problems that have plagued Dan throughout his postaccident life: diffuse axial injury, intermittent explosive disorder, anosognosia, aphasia, dysphagia, and dysarthria, as well as the infantilization, ostracism, exclusion, rejection, and bullying that followed in their wake. I better understand the crushing effects of loneliness and the life-affirming, lifesaving indispensability of belongingness. I have been able to explain to Dan's caregivers the inevitability of his IED episodes and to suggest strategies for dealing with them, which helped to lessen their frequency, intensity, and duration. Understanding that anosognosia and IED are common within the TBI population and are caused by neurological disruption, not immature willfulness or egoism, has helped those around him to expect these behaviors, better cope with them, and harbor less resentment toward him in their wake. Of course, both IED and anosognosia continue to cause difficulty—that's a given. But placing them within the context of TBI allows Dan's sociality, rather than his neurological impairments, to take center stage. As a result, he has been accepted and is even well-liked, behavioral explosions notwithstanding, within the Harbor community.

Fourth: *Active presence.* From the first moments of Dan's move to Harbor, I repeatedly emphasized to both Dan and his caregivers that I was always available by phone if a problem arose. In the early weeks and months, I received many phone calls, sometimes five or ten a day, but as Dan acclimated to Harbor and staff acclimated to him, the calls tapered off. I visited every day for the first six months or so, and together we addressed whatever problems arose. The care plan meetings offered at Harbor were invaluable, providing the time, space, and focus for everyone involved to discuss issues, ask and answer questions, relate information, and build positive partnerships.

As Dan gained familiarity with his new situation and the people involved in his care, and as he gained confidence in his ability to communicate with caregivers and they increased in their ability to understand him, he realized that he could satisfactorily manage most situations on his own. Still, he knows that he has my unconditional support, that I respect his autonomy and his right to make his own decisions (as long as no one's nose is within reach of his fist), and that I am willing to show up and stand beside him when he needs me. He knows that what's important to him is, for that very reason, also important to me.

I also ensured that Harbor personnel understood that I was not only an advocate for Dan, but I was also an advocate and resource for them. Without exception, I followed up and followed through. I explained Dan's perspective to his caregivers, but I also explained their perspectives to Dan. I helped him understand when his expectations were unrealistic. I worked to address issues by finding solutions that satisfied everyone involved. I sought to understand situations from all possible angles and to ensure that both Dan and Harbor staff knew that we all had the same aim: harmony, not autocratic control by anyone, over anyone.

Fifth: *Provision of activities.* When Carrie offered OBRA services that would get Dan out of the nursing home environment and into the Muncie community several times a week, I was thrilled; it was instantly clear to me that involvement in this program would literally change his life. And it did. Going out to lunch or to the movies gave variety, structure, and pleasure to his week. Finding other activities that he was both interested in and able to take part in wasn't easy, but when Carrie suggested therapeutic horseback riding as an outlet for Dan's longstanding love of horses, his eyes caught fire and the slate was set. All of these excursions greatly enriched his life, but sitting astride a horse again allowed him to reconnect with his pre-injury identity, and it brought him a measure of joy I don't think he expected to experience again.

Sixth: *Communication.* I make a point of encouraging Dan to share his thoughts and concerns with me so that he knows he's listened to and his perspective is taken seriously. Knowing we're understood is critically important to all of us, but because Dan has aphasia, conveying his thoughts and ideas is considerably more difficult. He often struggles to be understood, and he can never take for granted that he will succeed. Being understood therefore takes on broader and deeper dimensions for Dan. Time, patience, and a degree of guesswork are frequently required to suss out his meaning, and knowing what matters to him, what he thinks about, and his general frame of mind is helpful. When the people he deals with over the course of his day are pressed for time or patience, or don't have the right strain of imagination, or lack adequate familiarity with his perspective (and sometimes two or more of these factors together), Dan is often misunderstood. Sometimes people jump to conclusions, assuming they comprehend his thinking when they don't. Even those who diligently try to understand (including me) can't always grasp his meaning. I wrap up each of our phone calls with a simple but critical question: "Is there anything else you want to tell me before we hang up?" And if the answer is yes, I dedicate whatever time it takes for him to express it. Sometimes my understanding of what he's thinking seems to just snap into place, sometimes we struggle a bit before I arrive at it, and sometimes I just plain can't get there. And yet I believe that just honestly making the effort—prioritizing and doing our best to accommodate his need to communicate—profoundly matters, to both of us.

Two years in, the results have been staggering. Dan is, and always has been, uncommonly persevering, courageous, resilient, and optimistic. After years of feeling (and being) sidelined, he has reclaimed his life. He has become a valued member of the Harbor community, treated well by people who accept him, some of whom are genuinely fond of him. He has been woven into a mesh of belonging, which is what we all need most. When I recently asked him, "Your life is pretty good now, isn't it? Not perfect, of course—but good?" he smiled broadly and nodded.

★ ★ ★

A photograph taken at our parents' house less than a year following Dan's accident shows him standing ramrod straight, pronged cane in hand as a precautionary measure should he need the support. A truly handsome young man, he is neatly dressed in cream-colored khakis and a dark gold polo shirt that smartly contrasts with his wavy brown hair. Clear-eyed and slim, he regards the camera with a relaxed and open smile.

And yet, at the time, I barely saw his youthful vitality and striking good looks. The impressive qualities he still retained, the gains he'd already accomplished, the aspirations he still held—all were overshadowed by that cane. For me, the cane was less a tool that bolstered his balance and helped him walk than an insistent symbol of the impairment that had derailed his young life. All I could see or sense was loss and devastation. Indeed, there was plenty of that; repeatedly over the years, his injury was freshly traumatic in new and previously unimagined ways. But also, all along, there was the singular beauty and strength Dan still possessed, and possesses still.

I have learned at last to focus on the glittering smile, not the cane.

★ ★ ★

While I was writing this book, a memory resurfaced from the time of Dan's hospitalization in Tulsa, in the first few weeks after his accident. The families of brain-injured patients at St. Jude's organically formed a tightly knit community, because the shocking impact of TBI ravaging their sons or daughters, brothers or sisters, mothers or fathers, left them needing the support and understanding of others who were also experiencing it. Within this forlorn but desperately necessary little community, I met the parents of a boy roughly Dan's age who had been brain-injured in a motorcycle accident the year before. Eric remained comatose. Because doctors had told us that at least some people in Eric's (and Dan's) condition could hear and understand what was said to or around them, each day for the remainder of my stay in Tulsa, I visited Eric to offer encouragement. (I was only twenty-two years old, naïve, and new to the TBI phenomenon, believing with all the will I could muster that where there was life, there was hope.)

Photos of Eric taped to the walls around his bed displayed an adolescent boy who was cute by any standards. Tall and lean but athletically muscled like the surfer he had been, he had intelligent, friendly blue eyes below a swoop of blond hair, and his smile was toothy and engaging. The Eric on the hospital bed bore little resemblance to the boy in those pictures. His dark blond hair lay lank and damp nearly to his shoulders. His eyes were two slits, open about a quarter of an inch and staring blankly, which I mistook as an indication of the beginning of slow but impending emergence from his coma. Nude except for a sheet folded down to his waist, he was achingly emaciated, ribs standing in stark relief, diaphragm pumping like a bellows. His arms were little more than bones encased in skin, and both forearms angled upward across his chest, wrists turned severely inward so that the backs of his hands touched, contorted fingers forming tight, awkward fists on his collarbone.

And yet, I thought to myself (because I had to), where there's life, there's hope. Each day I spoke to him with a fervor that sounded like prayer, bubbling up with all the desperation I felt for Dan's recovery. But just before I had burned through the last of my two weeks of vacation days and had to return to my job in Fresno, Eric died. I began to wonder, although I admitted it to no one, if death was likely the best outcome for Eric and his family. And I feared, although I acknowledged this alarm not even to myself, that Dan might share Eric's fate, reduced to a breathing cadaver over the course of a year, until he finally died. It was several years before I was able to admit (and I was shocked to discover) that I suspected it would have been better for Dan if his accident had killed him too.

But I was wrong.

I was wrong even though Dan had to relearn *everything*—how to stand, how to walk, how to eat, how to brush his teeth, how to shave—and then lost some of those abilities, as well as some others, over the passing years. Even though he would never speak another word. Even though he was denied the pleasures of dating, of becoming a boyfriend, a husband, a father, a grandfather. And more. So much more.

I was wrong because Dan did, in fact, make a life for himself. It wasn't the life he had planned before the accident, but neither was his life irremediably ruined. Dan refused ruination—not by overcoming his impairments, but by optimizing his gifts, among which are his courage and resilience, his optimism, his indomitable sense of humor, and his capacity for love. Rather than endlessly loop through what he had lost, he concentrated on what remained and made the most of it. And four decades later, he still does.

For years, Dan's TBI was an open wound for *me*, and without conscious acknowledgment, I imposed distance between us in an effort to avoid the pain of it. But there was no escape. It wound even through my dreams, especially a surprisingly vivid recurrent one in which, under a past-midnight moon-shimmered sky with scudding black clouds, I pulled Dan, unconscious, from the lapping black waters of a bay onto a pier. His body was wet and cold, torn and bruised, and I held him in my arms, anguished. Like a movie camera, in this dream, my viewpoint shifted to above the scene to see us looking, for all the world, like Mary holding the ravaged dead body of Jesus. I drank quantities of wine every night after work, sometimes fruitlessly railing at a God I had never been quite able to believe in, but which I needed now to blame. I enlisted in the Navy in desperation, believing that separating myself geographically would separate me from my suffering and my emotional dysfunction. It didn't. I carried the wound with me for decades, still ragged at the edges, still painful to the touch.

But the process of bringing Dan to Indiana and examining his life to write this book has led to an epiphany. Immersed in his life day to day, and having become acquainted with a body of knowledge that had yet to be understood at the time of his accident over forty years ago, I've realized how much worse his situation could have been, and I more fully appreciate how well he has managed despite the circumstances he has lived within. And I have also recognized the part that belongingness plays in making our lives not just endurable but enjoyable. Dan savors his life in no small measure because he knows he has the love of his family and others who care about him, who embrace him with genuine affection.

It's true that Dan has faced, and continues to face, hardships that I have long considered unendurable. And yet he *has* endured, *does* endure, confronting his challenges with courage, determination, and astonishing good spirits. Despite the impairments he still lives with, Dan has healed. It may not be apparent to strangers, but he is healthy and whole. Understanding that truth—living it with him—has healed me, too. Without question, and without being blinded to Dan's very real human frailties and imperfections and the frustrations they generate, I view my brother as a real-life hero. I finally recognize the young man who woke up from that coma and took on every challenge that confronted him. I have finally gotten to know, and greatly admire, the man he has been and the man he has become.

At least as much as anyone else, Dan deserves acceptance, appreciation, and, above all, belonging.

Notes

1. Robert H. Kimball, "A Plea for Pity" *Philosophy and Rhetoric* 37, no. 4 (2004): 301–16, 304. doi: 10.1353/par.2004.0029
2. Kipling D. Williams, Joseph P. Forgas, and William von Hippel, *The Social Outcast: Ostracism, Social Exclusion, Rejection, and Bullying* (New York: Psychology Press, 2014); and Kelly-Ann Allen, *The Psychology of Belonging* (London: Routledge, Taylor & Francis Group, 2021).
3. Creigh Farinas, "Don't Call My Sister 'Cute'—6 Good Reasons to Stop Infantilizing Disabled People" *everydayfeminism* (December 5, 2015). https://everydayfeminism.com/2015/12/infantilizing-disabled-people
4. Matthew D. Lieberman, *Social: Why Our Brains Are Wired to Connect* (New York: Crown Publishing, 2013); Naomi Eisenberger, et al., "Does Rejection Hurt? An fMRI Study of Social Exclusion" *Science* 392, no. 5643 (2003): 290–2. doi: 10.1126/science.1089134; and Adnan Bashir Bhatti and Nawar ul Haq, "The Pathophysiology of Perceived Social Isolation: Effects on Health and Mortality" *Cureus* 9, no. 1 (2017): e994. doi: 10.7759/cureus.994
5. Kipling D. Williams, Joseph P. Forgas, and William von Hippel, "Introduction," in *The Social Outcast: Ostracism, Social Exclusion, Rejection, and Bullying* (New York: Psychology Press, 2014), ii.

11 Epilogue

Across the globe, the coronavirus that descended in 2020 changed everything, including Dan's situation.

On March 11, 2020, Harbor Health locked down. No one except staff could enter the building, and no one except staff could leave. Suddenly Dan could no longer go on outings for lunch, movies, or (most significantly) horseback riding. Suddenly I could no longer visit. Like nursing homes all over the country, Harbor became critically short-staffed and turnover was continual, and I couldn't be present to help introduce Dan to new personnel, to liaise with them, or to fill in whatever gaps developed. A few employees stayed with Harbor over the long haul, but none of them were Dan's nurses or CNAs. Due to critical staffing shortages, Harbor was forced to hire whomever they could get, and the quality of Dan's care—and consequently his quality of life—plummeted. Dan had gone from being mostly understood and appreciated to unknown and universally underestimated, despite my efforts to correct misapprehensions over the phone. My repeated pleas for staff to apply his elbow and wrist braces daily went unheeded, and the extreme contractures of his elbow, wrist, fingers, and thumb, which had taken months to improve after his arrival at Harbor, returned. Without regular physical therapy, including my nonprofessional but helpful stretching of his neck muscles, his chin returned to the position of resting on his chest, head cocked to one side.

Still, Dan remained in surprisingly good spirits. We talked on the phone at least every evening, but he didn't repeatedly call throughout the day out of boredom, as I'd thought he might. His calls for my intervention with staff increased, but not unreasonably so. Weather and my health permitting, we had window visits twice a week, where Dan and I talked on our phones as we smiled at each other from opposite sides of a picture window. That contact was helpful for both of us, but by no means was it a satisfying substitute for the in-person visits we were both accustomed

DOI: 10.4324/9781003340294-11

to. Dan did what he could to exercise, every day spending hours—usually six or seven of them—propelling himself in his wheelchair, covering all the hallways in the facility, repeatedly circling through the building in an effort to cultivate strength in his left arm and leg. He did everything he could to maintain as much as he could. And he was, if only barely, getting by.

In the fall, Carrie, who had set Dan up with OBRA visits, suggested that he might prefer living in a waiver home, a house he would share with a couple of roommates and a few rotating staff members to provide care around the clock. I was intrigued—but also wary. Dan's experience with Carl in Atlanta had ended catastrophically, and I trembled at the possibility of recreating a similar situation. But Carrie assured me that Dan wouldn't be abandoned. The company that he would sign with to provide his housing and care would know in detail what his care demanded, and his situation would be monitored by the state to ensure that the company upheld state standards and fulfilled its contracted obligations to him. Also, this time I would be nearby to safeguard his well-being and ensure that any bumps or lapses were addressed. When I felt quite certain that such a move wouldn't lead him into a worse situation than he was in at Harbor (a bar that, by that time, was pretty low), I brought up the possibility with Dan on one of our window visits. It was as though a dense fog suddenly lifted and the sun broke through, madly shining. Dan had no trepidation, no reservations. Presented with the possibility, he wanted out of Harbor and into a home setting. Full stop.

We okayed the process with Carrie. She and a placement caseworker interviewed me for several hours in order to get an in-depth understanding of Dan's background, what he would need from caregivers, and the challenges he would present. I was elated by the extensive interviews, because they reduced the chances that anybody, on either side of the contractual equation, would be much surprised by anything in the wake of his transition from Harbor to a private home.

After four months of preparation and searching for a situation that would work for him, Dan moved out of Harbor into a pleasant house on a tranquil street in a quiet neighborhood. He has his own room, which he'll be outfitting with new bedroom furniture that he'll pick out himself—the first furniture he will ever have owned in his adult life. He'll soon be a member of the YMCA, where he'll use its indoor track for his "walks." (We hope to link up with Agape again, although last summer they retired a number of their horses, and none currently in their stable is capable of supporting an adult's weight.) He's been getting along well with staff, and he reports that he's receiving greater attention and care than he'd been given at Harbor, at least over the eighteen months following Shiloh's departure. I've shared Dan's backstory with his new caregivers, and all indications are that they enjoy him, despite the occasional IED episode. There are still some issues to iron out; for example, except for a night when Dyke and I took him out for dinner, he's yet to have an outing—including a trip to the barbershop, doctor, or dentist—due to staff shortages. But he's still much happier. I remain mindful that I believed Harbor to be the perfect place for him when he first moved there, and in the beginning it was. He had a very good life in that facility for almost two years—but he lived there for three. Similarly, there may be a future point at which, for some as yet unforeseen reason, his new home no longer fits him well, and he may want to relocate again. However, his caseworker told me that if a placement isn't going work, usually it's apparent early in the transition period. So far it seems very hopeful, but if Dan ever wants to move, the caseworker will help him find another home that he might like better.

For now, though, Dan is happy where he is. As I am writing this, he's been in his new home for two weeks today. Earlier this week, I asked him if the house felt like home yet, and he answered with a cheery grin and a nod. Undoubtedly there will be challenges ahead, but so far, so very good.

While Dan's story is by no means over—life is no fairy tale, and there can never truly be a "happily ever after"—the beginning of this latest episode seems a good place to close. Besides, Dan is expecting me at his place this afternoon. There are pictures, a jockey helmet, and a horseshoe waiting to be hung on his bedroom walls.

Bibliography

Allen, Kelly-Ann. *The Psychology of Belonging*. London: Routledge, Taylor & Francis Group, 2021.
Baumeister, Roy F., and Mark R. Leary. "The Need to Belong: Desire for Interpersonal Attachments as a Fundamental Human Motivation." *Psychological Bulletin* 117, no. 3 (1995): 497–529. doi: 10.1037/0033-2909.117.3.497
Bhatti, Adnan Bashir and Nawar ul Haq. "The Pathophysiology of Perceived Social Isolation: Effects on Health and Mortality." *Cureus* 9, no. 1 (2017): e994. doi: 10.7759/cureus.994
Cacioppo, John T. and William Patrick. *Loneliness: Human Nature and the Need for Social Connection*. New York: W.W. Norton & Company, 2008.
Eisenberger, Naomi I., Matthew D. Lieberman, and Kipling D. Williams. "Does Rejection Hurt? An fMRI Study of Social Exclusion." *Science* 392, no. 5643 (2003): 290–2. doi: 10.1126/science.1089134
Farinas, Creigh. "Don't Call My Sister 'Cute'—6 Good Reasons to Stop Infantilizing Disabled People." *everydayfeminism* (December 5, 2015). https://everydayfeminism.com/2015/12/infantalizing-disabled-people
Flamm, Hannah. *"They Want Docile": How Nursing Homes in the United States Overmedicate People with Dementia*. New York: Human Rights Watch, 2018.
"Get the Facts about TBI." *Centers for Disease Control and Prevention*. Centers for Disease Control and Prevention, March 21, 2022. www.cdc.gov/traumaticbraininjury/get_the_facts.html
Goffman, Erving. *Stigma: Notes on the Management of Spoiled Identity*. Englewood Cliffs, NJ: Prentice-Hall, 1963.
Harrison-Felix, Cynthia, Scott E. Kreider, Juan C. Arango-Lasprilla, Allen W. Brown, Marcel P. Dijkers, Flora M. Hammond, Stephanie A. Kolakowsky-Hayner, Chari Hirshson, Gale Whiteneck, and Nathan D. Zasler. "Life Expectancy Following Rehabilitation." *Journal of Head Trauma Rehabilitation* 27, no. 6 (November 2012). doi: 10.1097/htr.0b013e3182738010
Holder, Eric. "Attorney General Press Conference Transcript, November 4, 2013." www.justice.gov/opa/speech/attorney-general-eric-holder-delivers-remarks-johnson-johnson-press-conference
Kagan, Aura and Nina Simmons-Mackie. "Changing the Aphasia Narrative." *The ASHA Leader* 18, no. 11 (2013). doi: 10.1044/leader.fmp.18112013.6

Kimball, Robert H. "A Plea for Pity." *Philosophy and Rhetoric* 37, no. 4 (2004): 301–16, 304. doi: 10.1353/par.2004.0029

Lieberman, Matthew D. *Social: Why Our Brains Are Wired to Connect*. New York: Crown Publishing, 2013.

Lim, D. K. and R. Mahendran. "Risperidone and Megacolon." *Singapore Medical Journal* 43, no. 10 (October 2002): 530–32.

Lux, Warren E. "A Neuropsychiatric Perspective on Traumatic Brain Injury." *The Journal of Rehabilitation Research & Development* 44, no. 7 (2007): 951–62. doi: 10.1682/jrrd.2007.01.0009

MacDonald, Geoff and Mark R. Leary. "Why Does Social Exclusion Hurt? The Relationship between Social and Physical Pain." *Psychological Bulletin* 131, no. 2 (2005): 202–23. doi: 10.1037/0033-2909.131.2.202

"Megacolon: What Is It, Causes, Symptoms, Treatment, and More." *Osmosis from Elsevier.* www.osmosis.org/megacolon

"Moderate to Severe Traumatic Brain Injury Is a Lifelong Condition." *Centers for Disease Control and Prevention.* www.cdc.gov/traumaticbraininjury/pdf/moderate_to_severe_tbi_lifelong-a.pdf

Omnibus Budget Reconciliation Act of 1987, 100th Congress, Pub.L. 100–203, 101 Stat. 1330–160, Title IV(C), Sec. 1819. https://budgetcounsel.files.wordpress.com/2017/01/omnibus-budget-reconciliation-act-of-1987.pdf

Prigatano, Frank P. *Principles of Neuropsychological Rehabilitation*. New York: Oxford University Press, 1999.

"Report to Congress: Traumatic Brain Injury in the United States." *Centers for Disease Control and Prevention.* Centers for Disease Control and Prevention, January 22, 2016. www.cdc.gov/traumaticbraininjury/pubs/tbi_report_to_congress.html

Scanlan, Lawrence. *Wild About Horses: Our Timeless Passion for the Horse*. New York: HarperCollins, 2001.

"TBI Among Service Members and Veterans." *Centers for Disease Control and Prevention.* Centers for Disease Control and Prevention, July 26, 2022. www.cdc.gov/traumaticbraininjury/military/index.html

"TBI Data." *Centers for Disease Control and Prevention.* Centers for Disease Control and Prevention, March 21, 2022. www.cdc.gov/traumaticbraininjury/data/

"Traumatic Brain Injury: Department of Defense Special Report." *Legacy Homepage.* U.S. Department of Defense. https://dod.defense.gov/News/Special-Reports/0315_tbi/

Williams, Kipling D., Joseph P. Forgas, and William von Hippel. *The Social Outcast: Ostracism, Social Exclusion, Rejection, and Bullying*. New York: Psychology Press, 2014.

Index

acceptance *see* belonging
alienation xi, 16
"alphabetting" 46–7
anger *see* IED
anosognosia 48–50, 68, 69; and "overcoming" impairment 49–50, 124–5; as both positive and negative 171–2
aphasia 7, 46–8, 73, 106, 171, 172, 182

BABY 113, 139, 174; *see also* baby talk; *see also* infantilization
baby talk 47; *see also* BABY *and* infantilization
belonging and belongingness xi–xii, 52–53, 106, 139–40, 153, 178–9; and care providers 43, 108–9; and survival 16–17, 35–6, 87–8
bullying 16, 112, 159, 174, 178–9

chemical restraint 21, 88, 122
cognition/cognitive processing xi, 51, 139, 171
cognitive behavioral therapy (CBT) 111, 144, 160

diffuse axonal injury (DAI) 44, 76
disability v. impairment 173
dysarthria 46–8
dysphagia 33, 48, 69, 172

empathy v. pity 173
exclusion 16, 53, 87, 174, 175, 178–9

Goffman, Erving 77

hemiplegia 45, 171–2

impairment v. disability 173
inclusion *see* belonging
infantilization 174–8; *see also* BABY *and* baby talk
intermittent explosive disorder (IED) 50–1, 89, 107–8; triggers 76–7, 107–8, 132, 142, 180–1
isolation xi, 16, 48, 51

liminality 139–140
loneliness 16–17

narrative/story 109, 180
nonverbal communication/messaging 106–107
"normal" as an organizational category 113, 139–40, 172

Omnibus Budget and Reconciliation Act of 1987 (OBRA) 122
ostracism xi, 16, 173–174, 178, 178–9

pity v. empathy 173

rejection xi, 16, 51, 173–4, 175, 178–9
rugged individualism 49–50,

schizophrenia 20–1
social connection *see* belonging
social pain theory 178–9

TBI statistics x; and longevity 161–2

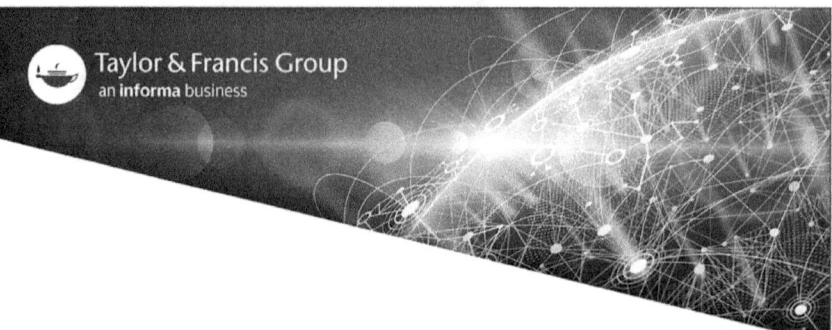

Taylor & Francis eBooks

www.taylorfrancis.com

A single destination for eBooks from Taylor & Francis with increased functionality and an improved user experience to meet the needs of our customers.

90,000+ eBooks of award-winning academic content in Humanities, Social Science, Science, Technology, Engineering, and Medical written by a global network of editors and authors.

TAYLOR & FRANCIS EBOOKS OFFERS:

- A streamlined experience for our library customers
- A single point of discovery for all of our eBook content
- Improved search and discovery of content at both book and chapter level

REQUEST A FREE TRIAL
support@taylorfrancis.com

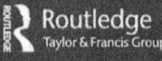 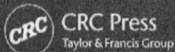

For Product Safety Concerns and Information please contact our EU representative GPSR@taylorandfrancis.com
Taylor & Francis Verlag GmbH, Kaufingerstraße 24, 80331 München, Germany

www.ingramcontent.com/pod-product-compliance
Lightning Source LLC
Chambersburg PA
CBHW051737230426
43670CB00012B/2058